Research Report

Challenges to the Sustainability of the U.S. Public Cord Blood System

Kandice A. Kapinos, Brian Briscombe, Tadeja Gračner,
Aaron Strong, Christopher Whaley, Emily Hoch,
Jakub P. Hlávka, Spencer R. Case, Peggy G. Chen

Sponsored by the U.S. Department of Health and Human Services

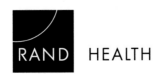

RAND HEALTH

For more information on this publication, visit www.rand.org/t/rr1898

Library of Congress Cataloging-in-Publication Data is available for this publication.

ISBN: 978-1-9774-0000-0

Published by the RAND Corporation, Santa Monica, Calif.

© Copyright 2017 RAND Corporation

RAND® is a registered trademark.

www.rand.org

Preface

In this report, we describe the existing public cord blood bank (CBB) system, assess current trends and economic relationships from the perspective of key stakeholders in the CBB system, and provide recommendations for ways to improve the economic sustainability of the system.

This report will be of interest to both private- and public-sector CBBs, health researchers, policymakers, and to other stakeholders of the CBB system, including pediatric and minority patients in need of transplants.

This research was sponsored by the U.S. Department of Health and Human Services, Office of the Assistant Secretary of Health under contract HHSP233201500038I, for which Rich Henry serves as the project officer. The research was conducted in RAND Health, a division of the RAND Corporation. A profile of RAND Health, abstracts of its publications, and ordering information can be found at www.rand.org/health.

Contents

Figures

Tables

Summary

Hematopoietic stem cells (HSCs)—from bone marrow, peripheral blood, or umbilical cord blood—are used to treat patients with cancers such as leukemia or lymphoma, disorders of the blood and immune systems, severe aplastic anemia, sickle cell disease, and certain inherited metabolic diseases.[1-3] Promising research also suggests a wide range of other possible applications of HSCs, including trauma repair, organ replacement, and treatment of more-prevalent conditions, such as diabetes or traumatic brain injury.[4-7] In addition to its direct therapeutic value to patients, cord blood is used for basic research on blood, blood stem cells, and immune cells.

There are several advantages and disadvantages to different HSC sources, and no single source is "best" in all circumstances for all patients. Although there are approximately 11 million individuals registered as bone marrow or peripheral stem cell donors in the United States, these sources require a stringent match to the patient and often require significant time, pain, and additional medical costs to collect donations. Cord blood stem cells are unique because they allow for less-precise matching of the donor's human leukocyte antigen (HLA) type to the recipient's HLA type. Evidence suggests that health outcomes from these less precisely matched cord blood cells are just as good as those from matched bone marrow grafts.[8] Cord blood is, therefore, particularly useful in cases where an exact match cannot be obtained from other sources—a situation which tends to occur more frequently in the United States for certain minority populations.[1] Cord blood collection also does not cause risk or pain to the mother or baby,[9] whereas bone marrow or peripheral blood collection is more invasive and imposes risks and discomfort to the donor. Cord blood collection typically occurs long before the units are needed, which means the units must be stored, usually for years, before they are used. However, the turnaround time between requesting a cord blood unit (CBU) and receiving it in a transplant center is generally very short in comparison with turnaround times for bone marrow and peripheral blood, which require extensive coordination with potential donors. On the other hand, the relatively small number of stem cells in cord blood compared with bone marrow or peripheral blood means the time for engraftment (i.e., the time required for the transplanted cells to take hold in the recipient's bone marrow and produce normal blood cells) is longer for cord blood.

In recent years, the U.S. government has endeavored to increase the overall national inventory of CBUs—which currently contains over 200,000 units—as well as the number of high-quality units and the number of units from racial/ethnic minorities. As we will describe in this report, these are two competing goals. The Stem Cell Therapeutic and Research Act of 2005[45] and the Stem Cell Therapeutic and Research Reauthorization Act of 2010[46] authorized the Secretary of the Department of Health and Human Services (HHS) to assist qualified cord blood banks (CBBs) with the collection and maintenance of the inventory goal of at least 150,000 new units of high-quality cord blood. The new CBUs were to be made available for transplantation through the C. W. Bill Young Cell Transplantation Program. The legislation and subsequent programs emerged due to an inability to recruit racial/ethnic minority adult donors to meet the clinical needs of a diverse U.S. population. In particular, some minority patients were historically unable to obtain other HSC units. Overall, the number of HSC transplants—which includes cord blood and other sources of HSCs—has increased over time, with 8,689 transplants taking place during fiscal year 2015, of which 718 transplants were cord blood. However, the percentage of HSC transplants using cord blood has declined over time, from about 12 percent (822) of all HSC transplants to about 8 percent (718) from 2010 to 2015.

The focus of this report is on the public banking system in the United States, which currently includes 19 public CBBs, and understanding factors related to future sustainability of the public system. Although we briefly discuss private CBBs, we only do so to the extent that their activities affect public CBBs. Therefore, unless otherwise specified, when we refer to CBBs, we mean public CBBs.

Although the federal government has been involved through regulating and subsidizing the public CBBs, we know little about the effects of government policies and funding arrangements on CBBs' financial outcomes and cord blood collection. Moreover, many public CBBs in the industry have reported significant financial stress and have expressed concern for the long-term trajectory of the industry, given current market conditions.

Despite the important clinical and research roles of cord blood products and a clear public health need for increasing and diversifying our national inventory, little is systematically known about the economics of the cord blood industry, including what banks' costs and revenues are, cost structures and determinants of financial health, successful collection efforts for CBBs, whether the market is competitive or similar to a public goods market, and the role of the government in the market.

In this report, we aim to fill these knowledge gaps by (1) describing the existing public CBB system, (2) assessing current trends and economic relationships from the perspective of key stakeholders in the public CBB system, and (3) providing recommendations to improve the economic sustainability of the public CBB system. For this report, cord blood system sustainability implies that there are enough public banks in the industry financially "breaking even" to maintain the current inventory as well as to increase the diversity and quality of the units collected in the future. In other words, we evaluate and propose changes that will improve the ability of public CBBs to cover their costs.

Key Findings

According to key stakeholders, the declining demand for CBUs is attributable to various forces, including an increase in the use of alternative sources of HSCs, the ongoing high costs of U.S. Food and Drug Administration licensure, and the medical challenges of successfully transplanting relatively small cord blood grafts compared with other HSC sources.

In our analysis of data from the National Marrow Donor Program (NMDP), which facilitates the vast majority of HSC transplants in the United States under the auspices of the HHS Health Resources and Services Administration (HRSA), we found a **decline in the proportion of HSC transplants that are cord blood, but a significant increase in the national cord blood inventory overall.** However, the growth in the inventory has been disproportionately concentrated among lower-quality (i.e., smaller) units.

In terms of quality, the total nucleated cell (TNC) count of a CBU is one of the most important measures used: Clinical guidelines recommend a minimum TNC count calibrated to patient weight and HRSA has established a TNC minimum for all CBUs added to the national inventory, which is called the Be The Match® Registry (hereafter, The Registry) and is maintained by the NMDP. Obtaining higher–TNC count units is costlier, but these units are significantly more likely to be used by patients. We found that about **half of the current national inventory is made up of CBUs that have TNC counts of less than 1.25 billion cells per unit, whereas the probability that a CBU with that cell count will be used in a given year is about one-tenth of a percent (or about an 11-percent chance that it will *ever* be used)** relative to a 1–3 percent chance that a CBU with a TNC of more than 1.5 billion will be used in a given year (or about a 61-percent chance that it will ever be used).

The TNC count also matters for increasing the racial/ethnic diversity of the national inventory. The federal government has prioritized increasing ethnic and racial minorities' access to cord blood. As noted above, a "less-precise" match is required for CBUs relative to other HSC sources, but this relationship between HLA-matching and patient outcomes is nonlinear and is affected by TNC count. Although an exact match is ideal, patient outcomes are statistically similar with one or two mismatched antigens *if* the CBU has a sufficiently large TNC count. Thus, **increasing racial/ethnic minority access to CBUs and increasing the diversity of the inventory can also be achieved, at least in part, by collecting higher–TNC count units.**

We investigated banks' costs of collection, testing, processing, storing, and releasing units as well as banks' revenues from transplants. On the patient side, we explored the evidence for the clinical benefits of cord blood transplants as well as how payments between transplant providers and payers typically occur, noting that the majority of cord blood transplants occurs in inpatient settings. This analysis allowed us to use an economic model to determine whether a public CBB participating in the National Cord Blood Inventory (NCBI) program would be able to cover their costs and break even. Our analysis suggests that **banks lose money on the collection of units with TNC counts of less than 1.5 billion.**

In addition to examining what is necessary for individual-level banks to remain economically viable, we calculated the total value to society—the value of having a readily available treatment option for conditions treated with cord blood. We found that **the social value far exceeds the social costs,** suggesting that, to the extent that the private market does not fully supply the inventory needed, government intervention could have economic justification. In particular, we estimated the annual societal benefit of having a national cord blood inventory to be around $1.7 billion relative to an annual cost of maintaining the inventory at about $60–70 million. Given that the federal government is already supporting the industry through the NCBI and other programs, we also considered alternatives to the current NCBI program. We discussed the advantages and disadvantages of the current subsidy structure, with recommendations for ways in which HRSA may better calibrate the program to meet the goals of increased diversity and quality of the national inventory.

Recommendations

Based on these findings, we make two main sets of recommendations to improve the sustainability of the U.S. cord blood system. The first set of recommendations pertains to the NCBI program, and the second set is relevant to the broader public cord blood system. We briefly summarize both sets here.

NCBI Program

HRSA should focus on efforts to **increase the diversity of the national inventory** by (1) providing funding that encourages banks to add collection sites where more minority CBUs can be collected or increasing subsidies for minority units, and (2) considering increasing the minimum TNC count threshold, especially for nonminority units. HRSA should also explore ways in which CBBs might specialize in the collection of different types of CBUs (e.g., minority versus Caucasian).

We discuss the trade-offs between increasing the TNC-count threshold and revising the way in which subsidies are paid. There are advantages and disadvantages to each approach, but we note that the current system incentivizes the banking of lower–TNC count units despite these units being the least-profitable units for banks. Thus, HRSA should consider these trade-offs in conjunction with the program objectives to modify the program so that the CBBs' efforts better align with the program goals.

HSRA should **standardize and consistently fund the NCBI contracts to the extent possible.** The uncertainty, both in terms of how the contracts will be funded as well as the frequency, results in market instability. CBBs are competing for NCBI subsidy contracts that may favor those CBBs that are financially stable, but do not contribute to diversity as much as other CBBs that may be less financially stable. Because HRSA might change which CBBs will have a contract for each fiscal year, this could contribute to the ability of CBBs to make long-term investments aimed at diversity that would take longer than a single fiscal year to establish.

Broader Recommendations for Public Cord Blood Banking

We also suggest other ways in which stakeholders can work together to strengthen different aspects of the industry by making changes to **payment, research funding, and knowledge sharing.** Payment could be structured similarly to the way organs are reimbursed, and although cord blood is costly to procure, there are other significant costs related to bone marrow and peripheral blood transplants that are often overlooked (i.e., costs to the donor and the cost of waiting to obtain units). We found a strong societal benefit to banking cord blood, quantified annually at about 2.5 times the cost of maintaining the system. As a result, we recommend continued federal support for cord blood stem cell research, despite discussions by cord blood researchers in our study that focus may be shifting away from cord blood research, given the growth in alternative approaches for HSC transplantation. Finally, we point out the advantages for sharing knowledge in the industry—especially if the overall cord blood industry does shrink—to avoid losing all clinical and technical knowledge specific to cord blood and cord blood transplantation.

Acknowledgments

The RAND Corporation team is grateful to all the key stakeholders who agreed to be interviewed formally, as well as several experts in academia and government who provided us with helpful contextual details about the industry. We are especially thankful to Karen Dodson, Michael Boo, and Arthur Busse at the National Marrow Donor Program, who provided us with critical data on banking, shipping, and financial aspects of the public sector. We would also like to thank all the people we interviewed for generously sharing their time and insights. We thank our quality assurance reviewers, including Mary Laughlin of the Cleveland Cord Blood Bank, and Shira Fischer, Peter Hussey, and Paul Koegel of RAND.

We especially thank our project officer, Rich Henry, for his guidance and review of the document. We note that the material contained in this report is the responsibility of the research team and does not necessarily reflect the beliefs or opinions of the project officer, the U.S. Department of Health and Human Services, the Office of the Assistant Secretary of Health, or the federal government.

Abbreviations

AABB	American Association of Blood Banks
AAP	American Academy of Pediatrics
ACOG	American Academy of Obstetricians and Gynecologists
AHRQ	Agency for Healthcare Research and Quality
ALL	acute lymphoblastic leukemia
AML	acute myelogenous leukemia
ANCTC	Anthony Nolan Cell Therapy Centre
APC	ambulatory payment classification
BLA	Biologics License Application
C	Celsius
C-APC	comprehensive ambulatory payment classification
CAR	chimeric antigen receptor
CBB	cord blood bank
CBU	cord blood unit
CDF	cumulative density function
CED	Coverage with Evidence Development
CEO	chief executive officer
CI	confidence interval
CIBMTR	Center for International Blood and Marrow Transplant Research
CMS	Centers for Medicare and Medicaid Services
DRG	diagnosis-related group
FACT	Foundation for the Accreditation of Cellular Therapy
FDA	U.S. Food and Drug Administration
FY	fiscal year
GAO	U.S. Government Accountability Office
GVHD	graft-versus-host disease

HCUP	Healthcare Cost and Utilization Project
HCUPnet	Healthcare Cost and Utilization Project online query tool
HHS	U.S. Department of Health and Human Services
HLA	human leukocyte antigen
HRSA	Health Resources and Services Administration
HSC	hematopoietic stem cell
ICD-9	International Classification of Diseases, Ninth Revision
IND	Investigational New Drug (application)
IPPS	Inpatient Prospective Payment System
kg	kilogram
MSC	mesenchymal stem cell
MS-DRG	Medicare Severity Diagnosis-Related Group
NCBI	National Cord Blood Inventory
NIS	National Inpatient Sample
NMDP	National Marrow Donor Program
OPPS	Outpatient Prospective Payment System
The Registry	Be The Match® Registry
Rh	Rhesus (group)
TNC	total nucleated cell
WMDA	World Marrow Donor Association

Chapter One. Introduction

Hematopoietic stem cells (HSCs) are derived from three distinct sources: bone marrow, peripheral blood, and umbilical cord blood (hereafter referred to as "cord blood"). HSCs are multipotent in that they have the potential to differentiate into several types of blood cells. After transplantation, HSCs create new bone marrow, which is the body's "factory" for producing red blood cells, white blood cells, and platelets. Transplanted HSCs can replace a patient's native bone marrow and go on to develop into normal, healthy blood-forming cells. Treatments using HSCs can be *autologous*, that is, used for the person from which the HSC originated, or *allogeneic* when used for a person other than the individual from whom it originated.

HSCs have been used to treat patients with cancers such as leukemia or lymphoma, disorders of the blood and immune systems, and certain inherited metabolic diseases. In addition, promising research suggests a wide range of other possible applications of HSCs, including trauma repair, organ replacement, and treatment of more-prevalent conditions, such as diabetes or traumatic brain injury.[4–7]

HSC Transplants Have Increased, but Cord Blood Transplants Have Declined Over Time

In Figure 1.1, we present the number of HSC transplants over time by HSC type based on data from the National Marrow Donor Program (NMDP) (see Chapter Three for more information on the NMDP). The categories of HSCs are cord blood, haploidentical donor, other related donor, or unrelated donor. The latter three categories are all from bone marrow or other peripheral stem cell sources. The figure shows HSC transplants increasing over time, with 8,689 transplants during fiscal year (FY) 2015, but also shows the percentage of those that used cord blood declining from a high of 12 percent (822) of all HSC transplants in FY 2010 to about 8 percent (718) in FY 2015. These data further show that the decline in the use of cord blood mirrors the increased use of haploidentical transplants, which is a technique for transplanting related donors' bone marrow or peripheral blood with only a partial match. We discuss haploidentical transplants in greater detail in Chapter Two. Overall, the percentage of HSC transplants that use bone marrow or other peripheral stem cell sources (i.e., haploidentical donors or other related donors) has increased from about 42 percent to 45 percent, while the percentage of unrelated donors has remained relatively flat. A 2012 study of international banks showed a similar downward trend in the use of cord blood.[10]

Figure 1.1. Number of HSC Transplants Over Time, by Source

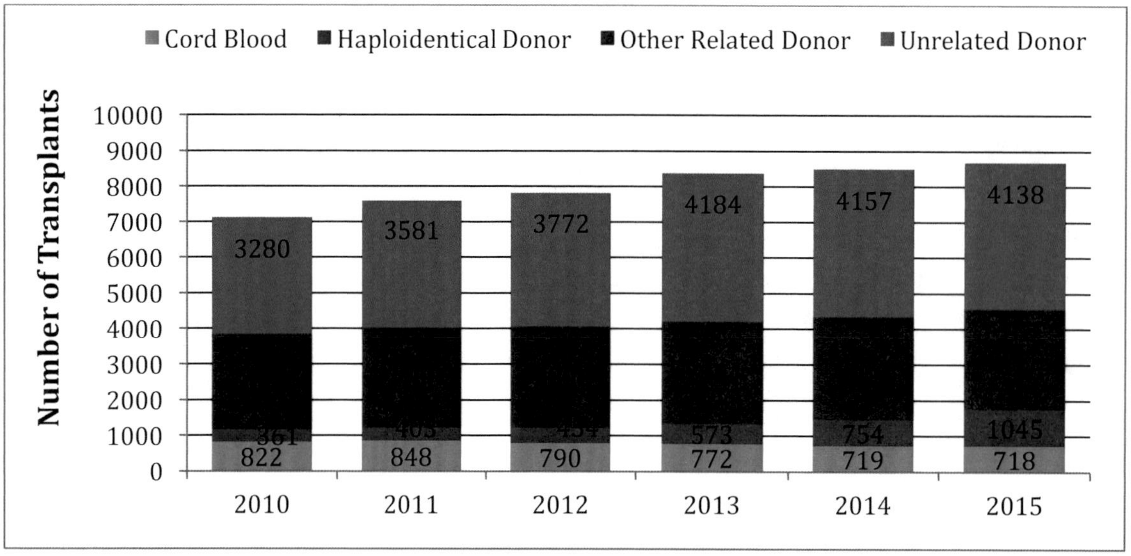

■ Cord Blood   ■ Haploidentical Donor   ■ Other Related Donor   ■ Unrelated Donor

Year	Unrelated Donor	Other Related / Haploidentical	Cord Blood
2010	3280	861	822
2011	3581		848
2012	3772		790
2013	4184	573	772
2014	4157	754	719
2015	4138	1045	718

SOURCE: NMDP Industry Shipment Data, 2010–2015.
NOTE: Categories of HSC source are mutually exclusive. Bone marrow and other peripheral stem cell transplants are included in three categories: haploidentical donor, other related donor, and unrelated donor.

Diseases Treated by HSC Transplants Are Rare, but Have High Mortality Rates

In Table 1.1, we present the number of transplants by the key conditions for which patients received HSC transplants in the United States from 2010 to 2016 based on data from the NMDP (see Chapter Three for more information). Overall, cord blood transplants represent only about 9 percent of all HSC transplants during this period. Although this is a relatively small percentage of HSC transplants, a closer look at the data helps to illuminate the patients likely to be affected by HSC-related policies, and cord blood–related policies in particular. For instance, the condition most frequently treated with HSC transplants is acute myelogenous leukemia (AML), with over 18,000 transplant patients, or 36 percent of all HSC transplant recipients from 2010 to 2016. AML is a cancer of the blood that primarily occurs in adults, with a median age of onset of 68 years.[11] Further, across HSC sources, AML accounts for a relatively stable one-third of all transplants. The next–most frequently treated disease using HSC transplants is acute lymphoblastic leukemia (ALL), accounting for 14.4 percent of all HSC transplant recipients. Like AML, ALL is a cancer of the blood. However, in contrast to AML, the median age of diagnosis for ALL is 15 years.[12] In addition, ALL accounts for 20 percent of cord blood transplants (1,002 out of 4,958) compared with 13–15 percent of transplants from other HSC sources.

Table 1.1. Number of HSC Transplants, by Source and Condition

Conditions	Cords	Haploidentical Donors	Other Related Donors	Unrelated Donors	All HSCs
Acute lymphoblastic leukemia	1,002	610	2,601	3,272	7,485
Acute myelogenous leukemia	1,777	1,536	6,139	9,359	18,811
Chronic myelogenous leukemia	109	161	565	826	1,661
Hodgkin lymphoma	82	160	430	522	1,194
Multiple myeloma	32	73	612	485	1,202
Myelodysplastic disorders	366	388	1,962	3,398	6,114
Non-Hodgkin lymphoma	351	437	2,102	2,441	5,331
Other disease, specify	20	16	43	67	146
Other leukemia	149	180	735	1,165	2,229
Other malignancy	118	162	778	1,217	2,275
Other nonmalignant disease	568	110	478	851	2,007
Primary immune deficiency	269	130	292	566	1,257
Severe aplastic anemia	58	107	773	709	1,647
Sickle cell disease	55	101	450	131	737
Total	4,958	4,171	17,960	25,009	

SOURCE: NMDP Industry Shipment Data, 2010–2016.
NOTE: Numbers represent the number of units shipped for transplant patients within a given condition. Categories of HSC source are mutually exclusive; see the Health Resources and Services Administration (HRSA) documentation for more details on disease categories.

Although the conditions for which HSC transplants are used with the greatest frequency are relatively rare, the conditions have high mortality rates and there are few options for treatment once patients experience disease recurrence after primary treatment. In 2017, an estimated 21,380 patients were diagnosed with AML, and just 5,970 patients were diagnosed with ALL. Although AML and ALL account for less than 3 percent of all cancers, they are associated with particularly high mortality rates and are the leading cause of cancer-related deaths in those younger than 39 years.[13, 14] In fact, the five-year survival rate for AML is just 26.9 percent. Thus, for a wide range of age groups, HSC transplants are a vital treatment for patients who do not attain remission of their diseases using other therapies.

Advantages and Disadvantages of Cord Blood

In HSC transplants, the donor's human leukocyte antigens (HLAs) need to match those of the recipient closely. There is wide diversity in human HLA types, and particularly in certain populations, such as African-Americans and Southern Europeans, who face greater challenges identifying HLA-matched HSC donors.[15] Current evidence indicates that just 25 to 30 percent of all patients will have an HLA-matched relative who can serve as a donor.[15] Patients who do not have an HLA-matched relative must then turn to unrelated donors, including individuals who have joined national registries for bone marrow or peripheral blood donations and public cord blood banks (CBBs) that store cord blood units (CBUs) for potential transplant.

However, research has demonstrated differences by racial/ethnic background in the ability to identify HLA-matched unrelated donors for bone marrow and peripheral blood.[16] In this study, although the majority of patients of Northwestern European or Eastern European ancestry and half of those of mixed European ancestry were able to find 10/10 HLA-matched unrelated bone marrow or peripheral blood donors, just one-third of those with Southern European ancestry, 19 percent of Asians, 8 percent of African-Americans, and 21 percent of Hispanic patients were able to find such a match (see text box). The availability of cord blood was noted to "extend stem cell availability to patients of both European and non-European origin" and findings demonstrated that more than half of cord blood transplant recipients were non-European.[16]

Text Box 1. Matching Donors with Patients: HLA Markers

The human body uses HLA genes to create a group of proteins known as the HLA Complex, which is found on the surface of most cells in the body. Individuals inherit half of their HLA genes from their mother and half from their father. Although HLA Complex proteins have a number of functions, one very important role is helping the body to distinguish the body's own cells from those that are "foreign" and that should be cleared from the body through an immune response. The best transplant outcomes occur when the components—or markers—of a patient's HLA Complex closely match those of the donor.

There are two classes of HLA markers: Class 1 and Class 2. Class 1 HLA markers are further classified into three types (A, B, and C) and Class 2 markers are further classified into six types (DP, DM, DOA, DOB, DQ, and DR). As an indication of the degree of diversity in the human genome, there are multiple forms of each HLA marker subtype (for example, there are at least 21 HLA type A antigens). Transplant centers typically examine at least eight HLA markers when looking for a match: two type A HLA markers, two type B HLA markers, two type C HLA markers, and two type DRB1 HLA markers. Sometimes an additional two type DQ HLA markers are also tested.[17, 18] The match is expressed as a ratio: For example, a 6/8 HLA-matched unit means that six out of the eight markers were the same in the patient and the donor. Many more markers can—and sometimes are— tested, but these are the most common.

A major benefit of cord blood is that it has less-stringent HLA-matching requirements compared with bone marrow and peripheral blood. Further, evidence suggests that health outcomes even from mismatched cord blood cells are comparable to those from matched bone marrow grafts.[8, 19] Once identified in a bank, cord blood is immediately available, unlike a donor, who may be difficult to locate or unable or unwilling to donate. However, as we have previously mentioned, CBUs are small relative to bone marrow and peripheral blood, meaning a longer engraftment period for cord blood transplants. Further, cord blood only provides a one-time source of HSCs—once the cells have been collected from a given donor, it is not possible to return to the same source to collect additional cells, as can be done with bone marrow or peripheral blood. Finally, because cord blood comes from newborn infants who have not had prior exposure to viruses, it does not impart any immune protection from prior viral exposures, as peripheral blood and bone marrow do.

Table 1.2 describes the various HSC sources, along with some relative advantages and disadvantages of each source. We note that future innovations may change the balance of these advantages and disadvantages. We will address the potential effects of innovations currently under investigation in Chapter Seven. Although a systematic review is beyond the scope of this study, we highlight key differences in clinical outcomes in the cost-effectiveness literature in Chapter Five.

Table 1.2. HSC Sources, Advantages, and Limitations

	Cord Blood Stem Cells	Adult Sources
Source	Umbilical cord blood following a healthy singleton birth.	Bone marrow (from a surgical procedure) or peripheral blood (nonsurgical, but requires premedication to stimulate stem cell release; long collection process, often eight or more hours).
Advantages	• Young cells, broad range of proliferation and differentiation capabilities • Readily available once collected and stored • Less-stringent HLA-matching requirements • Lower risk of GVHD infection than adult sources • Associated with lower relapse rates	• Maintain the ability to differentiate • Rich concentration of stem cells resulting in more-rapid engraftment • Can be harvested more than once • Extensive historical data for use • Transmits some immune protection from donor to recipient from prior viral exposure
Limitations	• Delayed short-term engraftment • One-time supply • Costly to procure, process, and store compared with other HSC sources • Lower volume of cells than adult sources unless double units or cell expansion technologies are used • Confer limited protection from prior viral exposure	• Less developmental potential compared with cord blood • Donor discomfort during harvesting procedure • Can take time to locate donor and schedule donation • Greater potential for GVHD than cord blood

SOURCE: Adapted from "A Comparison of Stem Cell Sources: Key Differences in Therapeutic Viability and Effectiveness."[20]
GVHD = graft-versus-host disease.

Some Public CBBs Are Struggling Financially to Cover Cord Blood Operations

Recent trends in the use of cord blood have had an impact on the potential future sustainability of public CBBs. A 2015 investigation by the World Marrow Donor Association (WMDA) found that only 11 percent of public CBBs worldwide are financially breaking even. According to the U.S. Government Accountability Office (GAO), CBBs in the United States have reported numerous financial challenges.[1, 21] Overall, the demand for cord blood in the United States has stagnated and there is considerable uncertainty about future projections of cord blood demand, which we discuss in more detail in subsequent chapters. Some have suggested that collection costs have increased as banks have been tasked with collecting CBUs from a more racially and ethnically diverse set of donors. As we discuss, key stakeholders report that obtaining licensure through the U.S. Food and Drug Administration's (FDA's) Biologics License Application, which the HRSA now requires for public CBBs, is costly. Because of the wide HLA diversity in the U.S. population, a relatively large number of CBUs representing a wide variety of HLA types must be banked to have sufficient inventory to draw on to identify matches for diverse patient populations. Yet CBBs must also collect and store inventory for years without any assurance that their inventories will be used. Furthermore, CBBs only receive the fee from transplant centers when a unit is withdrawn for use, which could be years after it was collected.

In addition to its direct therapeutic value to patients, cord blood is used for basic research on blood, blood stem cells, and immune cells. Despite the important clinical and research roles of cord blood products and a clear public health need for increasing and diversifying our national inventory, we know little about the economics of the public cord blood industry, including what banks' costs and revenues are, cost structures and determinants of financial health, successful collection efforts for cord blood banks, whether the market is competitive or more similar to a public goods market, and the role of the government in the market. Although the federal government has been involved through regulations and subsidies, we know little about the impact such policies and funding arrangements have on both CBBs' financial outcomes and cord blood collection.

Note that the focus of this report is on the public cord blood banking system in the United States and understanding factors related to future sustainability of the public system. Although we briefly discuss private CBBs, we only do so to the extent that their activities affect public CBBs. Similarly, we briefly discuss the international market, which clearly affects the U.S. market. Therefore, unless otherwise specified, when we refer to CBBs, we mean public CBBs.

Amid concern about the financial sustainability of the public CBBs in the industry, we aim to (1) describe the existing CBB system, (2) assess current trends and economic relationships from the perspective of key stakeholders, and (3) provide recommendations for ways to improve the system. Financial sustainability implies that there are enough banks in the industry "breaking even" to maintain the current inventory and to increase the diversity and quality of the units collected in the future.

To achieve these aims, we focus on the following key research questions in subsequent chapters:

- What are the current trends and challenges to public CBBs perceived by key stakeholders? (Chapter Four)
- What are the economic characteristics of the public cord blood market? (Chapters Five and Six)
- What is needed for financial sustainability? What is the market equilibrium? (Chapter Seven)
- What future developments might change the market? (Chapter Eight)
- What is the government's role in sustaining the industry and meeting society's needs? (Chapter Nine)

To answer these questions, we utilized a mixed-methods approach, drawing on both qualitative and quantitative research methods. We describe the details of our analytic approach in Chapter Three; briefly, we rely on (1) an environmental scan and review of pertinent literature, (2) semi-structured interviews with key stakeholders, and (3) an analysis of multiple data sources. This analysis is grounded in economics, health policy, and clinical practice.

Organization of This Report

The remainder of the report is organized as follows: In Chapter Two, we describe the current state of the U.S. public cord blood banking system, including key stakeholders, steps in the donor-to-transplant-recipient process, and key stresses on the system. This chapter is intended to serve as a primer for those unfamiliar with the structure of the cord blood system and to set the stage for later chapters where we aim to answer more-specific questions about important economic aspects of the system that may be contributing to the current state of affairs. Chapter Three provides details of our analytic approach. In Chapter Four, we present current industry trends and challenges, as identified by our key stakeholders. Chapter Five describes the economic characteristics of the cord blood system and includes empirical evidence on industry trends based on cord blood banking and shipping data. Chapter Six provides greater details on the economic interactions in the market, while Chapter Seven delineates the *profit-maximizing equilibrium*—the quantity and type of units to be collected given certain prices and costs for CBBs to cover their costs. In Chapter Eight, we discuss potential developments that could alter the cord blood market. Chapter Nine contains details on assessing the social value of the cord

In this chapter, we provide a brief overview of the cord blood system in the United States from donation to use, focusing on the actors and processes. We also describe the organizations involved and the regulatory and policy context in which they operate. This chapter is intended for readers who may not already be familiar with the U.S. cord blood system.

The Cord Blood Market

Cord blood is one source of HSCs, the others being bone marrow and peripheral blood. Thus, the cord blood market is part of a larger market for HSCs. Because cord blood is donated, the market is unique in that it does not pay donors. Public CBBs compete not only with one another to provide cord blood to transplant centers, but with other HSC sources, such as bone marrow and peripheral blood. When selecting the most appropriate source of HSCs, transplant centers weigh a variety of factors, including patient disease stage, patient comorbidities, prior treatments, the level of HLA match between donor and recipient, and timing and availability of the HSC sources. Importantly, bone marrow and peripheral blood are not banked—they are harvested from the donor for use by a specific recipient. Only cord blood is collected, processed, and banked in advance of any specific patient needing it. If the transplant center determines that cord blood is the best source of HSCs for a particular patient, the center must then choose the best CBU if there are multiple potential matches. As with selecting the most appropriate HSC source, choosing the best CBU is generally based on HLA profile, CBU size, and other factors, such as the CBB's reputation for quality and service.

Overview of the U.S. Public Cord Blood Banking System

If parents decide to donate their newborn's cord blood to a public CBB, the cord blood is collected following the delivery of the baby. Generally, public CBBs only collect cord blood from healthy singleton births. The collected cord blood is then tested for a variety of infectious diseases, assessed for general parameters indicating quality, and, if it passes these tests, is stored by the CBB and listed on the Be The Match® Registry (hereafter, The Registry), where it is available to any patient who needs it. Donors to public CBBs do not pay any fees to have their cord blood collected or stored. As of 2016, it is estimated that over 710,000 CBUs are currently available in public CBBs worldwide,[22] of which 235,000 are banked publicly in the United States.[23]

Figure 2.1 depicts the key stakeholders in the public cord blood banking system in the United States: CBBs, the hospitals and physicians with whom they coordinate collection and transplantation, payers, and several government agencies that facilitate both the collection and banking of cord blood (e.g., HRSA) and oversee the safety of the system (e.g., the FDA). Figure 2.2 outlines the key steps of cord blood collection, testing, processing, and storage, and we further analyze these processes in later chapters. We organize the discussion of the system by key steps in the process and with discussions of the key stakeholders within each section.

Figure 2.1. Key Stakeholders in the Current Public Cord Blood Banking System in the United States

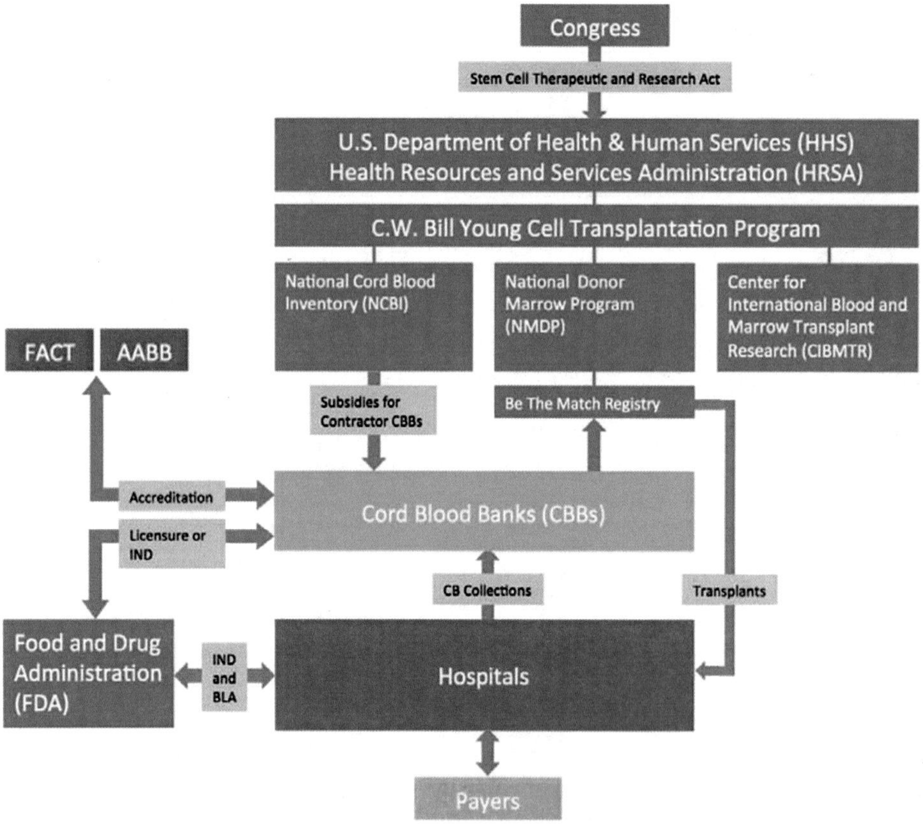

NOTES: AABB = American Association of Blood Banks. BLA = Biologics License Application. CB = cord blood. FACT = Foundation for the Accreditation of Cellular Therapy. IND = Investigational New Drug (application). Boxes in blue denote U.S. government agencies or programs. Payers include both private and public payers.

Text Box 2. Private (Family) Cord Blood Banking

As an alternative to public cord blood banking, individuals may pay a private CBB to bank their newborn's cord blood for their family's own use. This is called *family banking* or *private cord blood banking*. In private banking, individuals pay a collection fee as well as either an annual or lump-sum storage fee. CBUs in a private bank are only available to the family that deposited them. As of 2014, one report estimated that approximately 4 million CBUs had been privately banked worldwide, including 1.26 million banked in the United States.[25] We note that the American Academy of Pediatrics (AAP) recommends public banking and discourages private banking for most families. Research suggests that transplant physicians are reluctant to use privately banked CBUs[26] and several experts in the field have made arguments against private banking. A review of this literature is beyond the scope of this study, but we note that hybrid models of cord blood banking were mentioned in several interviews (and have been studied elsewhere).[27]

Private CBBs produce marketing materials targeted to expectant parents and some pay obstetricians to recommend their bank specifically. Typically, private CBBs can collect CBUs from any hospital in which an obstetrician or midwife is willing to perform the collection. They do not typically employ their own staff to collect cord blood.

Private banks are regulated differently than public CBBs and operate under very different market conditions. Private banks are not required to hold FDA licensure or to hold accreditation, although some do voluntarily. Private CBBs, like public CBBs, do need to *register* with the FDA, which involves providing a list of every blood product manufactured, prepared, or processed for commercial distribution twice per year.[28] Private CBBs are also required to adhere to current "good tissue practice" regulations and to conduct donor screening and testing for infectious diseases (except when cord blood is used for the original donor). Some private CBBs contract with other private CBBs—or even public CBBs—to process and store CBUs. In any private–public CBB arrangement, CBUs from private CBBs must be processed and stored separately from those from the public CBBs, in compliance with federal regulations.

This report focuses on the public cord blood system. Our discussions refer to private CBBs only to the extent that they affect the public cord blood market. Throughout this report, *cord blood banking* refers to public CBBs unless specifically noted.

Figure 2.2. Overview of Cord Blood Collection, Testing, Processing, Storage, and Use in the United States

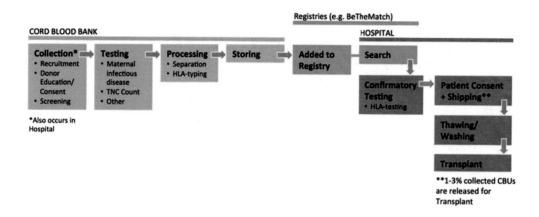

NOTE: TNC = total nucleated cell. Authors' interpretation and adaptation of Figure 4-1 from the Institute of Medicine[24].

Recruitment and Donor Education

Public CBBs are required to process and store collected units within 48 hours of collection (in keeping with accreditation and regulatory requirements). Thus, collection efforts tend to occur in geographically proximate hospitals, with a few notable exceptions. Currently, public cord blood banking is available in fewer than 200 hospitals in the United States.[29] This, coupled with the lack of funding for marketing campaigns, means that recruitment and education of expectant parents provided by public CBBs is typically minimal, mostly consisting of websites to provide education and guidance to expectant parents who want to donate their baby's cord blood. Most public CBBs rely on hospital volunteers (including physicians, prenatal class instructors, and labor and delivery nurses) to encourage expectant parents to donate, provide information about donation, and to collect the cord blood at the time of delivery. Some public CBBs maintain their own staff in collection hospitals to provide information and education about cord blood donation or consent-and-obtain information for the maternal questionnaire. Other parents learn about public cord blood banking through family and friends, while still others may learn about it through pamphlets or brochures from obstetricians and pediatricians. Finally, many states have laws requiring obstetricians to inform their patients about cord blood banking.[30] However, most legislation does not specify whether public or private donation should be discussed.

Cord Blood Collection, Processing, and Storage

Families who decide to donate their newborn's cord blood to a public CBB must provide a maternal health history and a maternal blood sample for infectious disease screening prior to delivery. Results indicating the presence of infectious disease must be reported to the patient's state health department.[31]

As previously discussed, the majority of public CBBs rely on hospital volunteers for recruitment, education, and collection efforts. Some public CBBs have on-site staff for recruitment, education, and maternal screening, and just a few public CBBs hire their own staff to perform cord blood collections.

There are advantages and disadvantages to each approach. Relying on hospital volunteers is inexpensive for CBBs and capitalizes on ongoing relationships between hospital staff and patients to encourage cord blood donation. In fact, existing research coupled with our own interviews of public CBB representatives indicates that the most-effective recruitment method for public CBBs is education and encouragement from hospital staff.[32] However, this approach can leave cord blood collections vulnerable to variations in collection practices and, therefore, variations in the quality of the collected cord blood. Employing CBB staff to provide in-hospital information and education and to guide women through consent and the maternal questionnaire is costly, but can also help improve precollection screening to optimize quality in collected cord blood. However, since hospital volunteers still perform the actual cord blood collection, there may be challenges with variations in collection practices between collectors. Employing CBB staff to perform collections is the costliest approach and also limits the number of collections, since CBB staff are only present during certain hours compared with hospital staff and physicians, who are required to be present at all deliveries. However, interviews with representatives from public CBBs who use this approach indicate higher TNC counts among collected units, translating to a lower rate of discarded CBUs. This was attributed to greater expertise and consistency among cord blood collectors.

In Figure 2.2, we describe the various steps involved with collecting, testing, processing, storing, and later withdrawing cord blood from a public CBB. In general, most banks collect cord blood in a sterile storage bag containing an anticoagulant.[25, 24] Collected cord blood is then packed, stored, and transported, typically in a temperature-monitored environment, to a cell-processing laboratory. While in transit from the collection site to the processing and storage site, time and temperature affect the viability of the cord blood: One study reported a 1-percent drop in cell viability for every 4-hour increase in transit time.[33]

After collection, but before further testing or processing, many public CBBs perform an initial assessment of the collected unit to determine its weight and volume. Low-weight or -volume units are usually discarded or donated to research at this time, since they are unlikely to meet minimum cell count requirements for banking and use in transplants given current technology.

On arrival at the CBB, CBUs undergo a variety of tests. Public CBBs largely submit to standardized testing to determine the volume by weight, the HLA type, and the quality (generally based on TNC counts, number of colony-forming units, and/or CD34+ [a protein found on the surface of the cell] counts). Additionally, banks may conduct screening for bacterial, viral, and fungal contamination.

Table 2.1 indicates the types of testing that public CBBs may order on the maternal blood sample and the CBU.[34–36] Some of these tests, particularly testing to ensure that infections are not transmitted from donor to recipient through cord blood, are required by the FDA. Other tests, while not required, are performed in some form by all public CBBs, given the need to determine the viability of the cord blood sample and ensure appropriate matching.

If the sample passes this step of the review, most banks remove red blood cells and plasma from the CBU.[25] Most banks also cryopreserve the cord blood using controlled-rate freezing, most often 1°C per minute. The sample is typically stored in liquid nitrogen at temperatures of at least –150°C.[25, 9] Generally, a portion of the CBU is frozen separately to allow for later testing (i.e., if the unit is identified as a candidate for use).[24] In some cases, there is a follow-up conversation with the donor family to verify whether the infant was healthy and whether there were any complications following the birth for either the infant or mother. This may be done at the point of storage, or it may be done much later, when the CBU is withdrawn for use.[22]

Table 2.1. Potential Testing for CBUs

Test	Purpose	Maternal Blood	CBU
Matching tests			
HLA-typing	Determines match with potential recipients	X	X
ABO blood group and Rhesus (Rh) factor	Determines match with potential recipients		X
Hemoglobinopathy screening	Tests for problems with hemoglobin that may be passed on through cord blood transplant		X
Counting/viability tests			
TNC enumeration	Total number of stem cells present in the sample		X
CD34+ cell number	Additional test of number of stem cells in sample		X
Colony-forming unit assay	Test of the viability of cells in the sample		X
Infectious disease screening			
Bacterial infection screening[a]	Infection screening	X	X
If bacterial infection screen is positive: bacterial culture (for aerobic and anaerobic organisms)	Infection screening	X	X
Infectious disease testing[a] Cytomegalovirus, HIV, HTLV, hepatitis B, hepatitis C, syphilis, Chagas disease (maternal blood only), *Treponema pallidum*,[b] chlamydia, gonorrhea, West Nile Virus, Zika	Infection screening	X	X

NOTE: HIV = human immunodeficiency virus. HTLV = human T-lymphotropic virus.
[a] The FDA requires these tests.
[b] *T. pallidum* is a bacterium that causes syphilis.

At any point in the process, a CBU may be identified as unsuitable for storage for any number of reasons, including low volume (i.e., not enough stem cells to use in a transplant), poor viability (i.e., there may be stem cells, but they may not be alive or appropriately functioning), poor results from infectious disease testing, or negative findings from the maternal health questionnaire. Some evidence indicates that for every 100 births otherwise eligible for cord blood donation (that is, births with no exclusionary conditions, such as multiple gestations, premature birth, or other maternal or child health conditions that preclude donation) in which cord blood collection is attempted, 45 CBUs are sent for processing and only ten are ultimately stored.[37] This information corroborates reports from key stakeholders representing public CBBs in this study, who indicated that anywhere from 10–30 percent of collected CBUs were ultimately stored.

Cord Blood Inventory Management and Withdrawal

Logistics and Inventory Management

Most cord blood stored in public banks in the United States is listed with NMDP, which runs The Registry and serves as a "one-stop shop" for patients seeking HSC transplants of all kinds. Many international banks' cord blood is also available through The Registry.

Some public CBBs may also offer units that do not meet qualifications for being listed on The Registry, but may still have value to potential recipients (e.g., they may have lower cell counts, but represent rare HLA types). These are not available through The Registry, but rather are obtained directly through established relationships with CBBs.

Identifying a CBU for Transplant

When a patient has a condition that necessitates treatment using an allogeneic HSC transplant, the patient's physician, whether in the United States or abroad, can search existing registries, including The Registry, for a potential match. Cord blood from 19 public CBBs in the United States and five international banks, as well as registries in 39 countries, are listed on The Registry.[24, 38, 39] More than 90 percent of CBUs distributed for transplant in the United States are distributed through The Registry, which has a congressional mandate to serve as a single point of access that can be used to search for unrelated marrow donors and CBUs.[38, 40] The NMDP also facilitates financial transactions between CBBs and transplant centers for units that are listed on The Registry.[38] Finally, the availability of cord blood in international registries also helps increase the potential for a match. In 2012, the WMDA reported that over 4,000 CBUs were shipped for unrelated patients in 46 different countries.[10]

Most patients who require an HSC transplant will find a donor, whether the source required is bone marrow, peripheral blood, or cord blood.[40] However, depending on the patient's ethnicity, HLA profile, and other factors, the transplant center may receive a varying number of potential matches. The NMDP search yields a Preliminary Match Report that lists all potential HSC sources available (cord blood, peripheral blood, and bone marrow). Upon reviewing the report, the provider and patient can decide which available source is best. The discussion below focuses only on what happens if the transplant physician chooses a CBU as the source for transplant.

CBUs are sorted by the level of HLA match and TNC count (cells per kilogram [kg] of a patient's weight).[38] If a suitable CBU match is found, the physician or transplant center can request an Individual Match Report for each unit under consideration, which gives detailed information about the CBU; the HLA type; and measures of quality, such as the number of TNCs and CD34+ cells; tests for compatibility, such as ABO blood type and Rhesus blood group; as well other test results that were conducted prior to the CBU being stored. The report will also include some information from the medical history, potential risks for infectious or genetic diseases, and any other details that might affect the quality of the CBU. Typically, a CBB will also request a blood sample from the transplant recipient to confirm that the HLA type of the patient matches the HLA type of the CBU. In addition, transplant centers can request samples of the CBU to conduct special testing—for instance, to measure enzyme levels for specific genetic diseases or for infectious agents that are not part of routine testing. Generally, prior to storage, a small aliquot is frozen separately so that the entire CBU does not need to be thawed to conduct such testing.

Once the most appropriate HSC transplant graft is selected, the transplant physician completes a formal request form documenting that he or she has reviewed the information provided and approves the transplant.

Requested CBUs are shipped to the transplant center, typically via overnight courier in a container that uses liquid nitrogen to maintain the temperature at −150°C. The temperature is monitored and documented continuously. There is variation across transplant centers in how they thaw and wash the CBUs, with some experts noting concern with the chain of custody and ultimate efficacy of a CBU.

Finally, we also note that many public CBBs provide CBUs for research purposes. In many cases, these units have not met the criteria for banking. In less-common cases, CBUs listed on registries for transplantation may be withdrawn for research purposes.

Transplant Procedure

For patients who have been deemed appropriate candidates for a cord blood transplant, there are several preparatory steps to undertake.[41] Most of these steps will be the same for any HSC transplant. Patients will generally receive a central venous catheter—also called a *central line*—which is a long, thin, flexible tube that is used to administer medicines, fluids, nutrients, or other treatments over time, usually several weeks or more. The catheter is usually inserted in the arm or chest, through the skin and into a large vein. Patients will also receive their transplant cells through the central line. In addition, since transplant patients need to have blood drawn for a variety of tests, a central line helps make the process more comfortable by eliminating the need for repeated punctures.

Patients also must undergo a conditioning regimen—also referred to as *purging*—which is the process of getting the body ready for transplant by destroying diseased cells in the body, destroying a patient's native bone marrow (to make room for the transplanted cells), and stopping the patient's immune system from functioning so that it does not recognize the transplanted cells as foreign. There are a variety of conditioning regimens of varying intensity and involving combinations of chemotherapy and/or radiation therapy, depending on the patient's specific circumstances.[42] Many patients who are eligible for a low-intensity conditioning regimen (meaning that the patient's own bone marrow is not completely eliminated) may even be able to receive their transplant without being admitted to the hospital. However, they will typically need to visit an outpatient clinic regularly, even daily, and may still be admitted if complications arise. Patients who undergo myeloablative, or high-intensity, conditioning will generally be admitted to the hospital because their own bone marrow is eradicated. These patients are usually admitted to a special section of the hospital for transplant patients, which helps minimize the risk of infection and other complications. It is also important to help ensure that the staff caring for transplant patients is experienced in this specialized aspect of patient care, particularly in recognizing early warning signs of potential complications.

Once the conditioning process is complete, the transplanted cells are infused through the central line. The number of cells, and thus the length of the infusion, depends on the patient's size, with smaller patients requiring a smaller number of transplanted cells. The period immediately following the transplant is called the *engraftment period*, which is the time in which the transplanted cells establish themselves in the patient's bone marrow. The engraftment period generally occurs between 25 and 42 days after transplant, which is slightly longer than the engraftment period for other sources of HSCs.[43] During the engraftment period, physicians and staff must exercise vigilance for infection and complications, such as GVHD. Engraftment is considered successful when a patient's blood cell counts begin to increase, indicating that the transplanted cells are working properly. This depends on several factors, including disease, conditioning treatment, and factors related to the transplanted unit.[44]

Cord Blood Regulations and Government Policies

Here we provide an overview of the different regulatory and accreditation bodies that affect public CBBs.

Congress and the Stem Cell Therapeutic and Research Act

The Stem Cell Therapeutic and Research Act of 2005 provided the initial funding for the "collection and maintenance of 150,000 new units of high-quality cord blood to be made available for transplantation through the C. W. Bill Young Cell Transplantation Program."[45] The Act authorized NCBI to receive an appropriation of $15 million in federal funds for each fiscal year, from FY 2007 through FY 2010, to help meet this goal. The Act's reauthorization in 2010 changed the NCBI language from 150,000 new units to "at least 150,000" units and allocated $23 million from FY 2011 through FY 2014 and

$20 million in FY 2015.[46] The 2015 reauthorization for the C. W. Bill Young Cell Transplantation Program provided an authorization of $30 million from FY 2016 to FY 2020.[47]

HRSA

HRSA administers the C. W. Bill Young Cell Transplantation Program and manages its various components. HRSA provides funding for the collection of diverse CBUs for NCBI through contracts to CBBs. There are 13 NCBI contractors who bid to provide a certain number of CBUs of certain types (e.g., racial/ethnic groups).[48] Despite its name, NCBI is not a separate registry. Rather, once NCBI-eligible CBUs are listed on The Registry, public CBBs receive a subsidy for cord blood collection, processing, and storage. This subsidy does not cover the entire costs borne by CBBs for collection, processing, and storage, but it does help defray some of those costs.

NMDP

The NMDP provides the link between HRSA, CBBs, and physicians for obtaining stem cells and, specifically, cord blood. The Registry provides physicians with software designed to find the best available stem cell candidates for the patient. The NMDP acts as the intermediary between the CBB and the transplant center once a CBU has been located. The NMDP also acts as the financial intermediary between individual CBBs and hospitals. The NMDP also provides education for patients and clinicians.

Accreditation Bodies

By law, all public CBBs must be accredited to ensure that they meet high quality and safety standards. The Secretary of HHS recognized the AABB and the FACT as accreditation entities for NCBI CBBs. Some private banks also choose to obtain accreditation.[45, 46, 49–51] The accreditation processes require CBBs to adhere to a set of quality standards meant to serve as minimal requirements with the expectation that CBBs should treat them as a "floor" not a "ceiling."[52, 53] There are some differences in accreditation between the two bodies. For instance, FACT accreditation addresses the thawing and washing process, while AABB does not.[54]

In addition, the WMDA offers accreditation to blood stem cell organizations, including registries. These activities are designed to help facilitate the search for unrelated donors for patients in need of a transplant.[55]

FDA Oversight

The FDA regulates cord blood in a variety of ways, depending on the source, the processing, and the intended use.

Cord blood stored in private banks (i.e., for autologous use or use in first- or second-degree relatives) does not need to go through FDA licensure because it is used on the individual from whom it was collected, or on a related individual. In contrast, public CBBs store CBUs intended for use by a patient unrelated to the donor (e.g., for allogeneic use). Therefore, this use meets the legal definitions of both a "drug" and a "biological product," which means that public CBBs must adhere to additional requirements. Public banks are required to comply with good tissue practice regulations, conduct specific donor screening and infectious disease testing (see Table 2.1), conduct standardized testing on CBUs, and maintain international cellular therapy accreditation. Potential donors must provide a health history and a maternal blood sample must be drawn within a week of delivery and screened for infectious diseases. Positive results must be reported to the state health department for the patient.[31]

Further, public CBBs are required to hold licensure from the FDA. This means that their CBUs must be licensed under a BLA that provides licensure for a large number of CBUs. The costs and time line for achieving FDA licensure are reportedly high, with many public CBBs reporting a 12- to 24-month timeline, initial costs of approximately $1 million, and ongoing annual costs of more than $100,000.[56–60] Despite a federal government requirement for public CBBs to hold FDA licensure, to date, only seven public CBBs have obtained FDA licensure.[61]

It is also important to note that individual CBUs are licensed, not the CBB itself. Since most public CBBs in the United States were in operation before the FDA licensure mandate—the FDA issued guidelines for licensure in 2009 and issued the first licensed product in 2011[62]—they have both licensed and unlicensed CBUs. *Licensed CBUs* are units meeting FDA standards, and *unlicensed CBUs* are units collected and processed prelicensure, or are postlicensure collections that do not meet the requirements specified by the FDA. Public CBBs that have not achieved FDA licensure will produce only unlicensed CBUs. Finally, CBUs from foreign CBBs are also unlicensed. The use of an unlicensed CBU must go through the process of an IND application.[63] An IND may be submitted by the manufacturer (the CBB), the transplant physician, the transplant center, a national or international cord blood registry involved in coordinating the distribution, or another qualified sponsor.[63] INDs are granted only for specific uses.[64] Bone marrow or other peripheral blood stem cells are not required to be licensed.

Related Research

Broadly, research utilizing cord blood can be categorized into (1) research utilizing CBUs in novel ways to treat human disease, and (2) research exploring ways to manipulate the CBU itself. Current studies are exploring the potential of cord blood for a variety of diseases, as described in Chapter One, as well as developing CBU expansion techniques and methods to optimize how CBUs are collected, processed, stored, washed, and thawed before being transfused.

Because public CBBs partner with specific hospitals to act as collection sites, women who deliver at other hospitals are typically not eligible for public cord blood banking. Some hospitals, particularly hospitals in academic research centers where research utilizing cord blood may be conducted, have procedures to retrieve these discarded cells and tissues for use in research. Institutions have varying policies around consent for collecting these discarded CBUs, with some requiring specific consent and others including it in their blanket consent for treatment.

Researchers can also request cord blood from public or private CBBs, and some CBBs have developed collaborations and partnerships with researchers in both academic medical centers and in privately held biotechnology firms. In some cases, researchers with specialized needs may be able to purchase CBUs already on The Registry from public CBBs, although this is uncommon and would be limited to smaller units that are unlikely to be used for transplant purposes. Because private CBBs are paid to collect, process, and store units, they do not have large numbers of discarded units to provide to researchers. According to an interviewer representing a private CBB, most private CBBs' discarded units are units for which families have stopped paying storage fees. For these units, private CBBs have also developed partnerships with private- and public-sector researchers.

Funding for cord blood–related research comes from a variety of sources. Private-sector research (i.e., research conducted by private organizations, such as biotechnology companies, laboratory testing companies, and other private companies providing supplies to the cord blood industry) is generally funded by the private sector itself. Public-sector research (i.e., research conducted in academic medical centers or other academic research settings) may be funded by government entities, such as the National Institutes of Health, or by private foundations and other philanthropic means.

In this chapter, we outline the overall analytic approach of this study, with a focus on the qualitative and quantitative data utilized. In Chapters Four to Eight, we provide more details and describe analytics unique to each chapter. We employed a mixed-methods approach, drawing on both qualitative and quantitative data from several sources. Our study was reviewed and approved by the RAND Human Subjects Protection Committee.

Literature Review

We reviewed the literature to gain an overall understanding of the public cord blood system and market in the United States and to inform our interviews and empirical analyses. We also surveyed the literature to help identify potential sources of quantitative and qualitative information on cord blood banking in the United States.

Our literature review encompassed both the peer-reviewed literature and grey literature (e.g., government reports, industry association reports, and other non–peer reviewed research). We reviewed articles for information on (1) the cost structures of CBBs; (2) payment models; (3) statistics and trends in the donation rates, diversity, and quality of units collected; (4) government regulations, funding, and other government involvement relevant to cord blood; and (5) current clinical practices related to cord blood.

Qualitative Approach

The goal of our qualitative data collection was to identify the challenges to and facilitators of a sustainable U.S. cord blood banking system. Specifically, our qualitative data collection comprised a series of semi-structured interviews with key stakeholders, including public and private CBB leaders and managers, transplant center physicians, representatives from relevant government agencies, researchers who utilize cord blood, and leaders of organizations that provide supplies for cord blood banking. We also interviewed representatives of private CBBs to understand the extent to which their activities affect public CBBs and the public cord blood banking industry.

We also sought input from various other stakeholders, including HRSA, the NMDP, the FDA, and other subject-matter experts who provided clarification, additional details, and contextual insights into the information we gathered from the literature.

Sampling

In identifying individuals to interview, we sought to achieve a wide range of perspectives within each respondent group. For public CBBs, we sought diversity along factors such as FDA licensure, racial and ethnic diversity of banked units, CBB size (i.e., number of units banked annually), and ownership structure (i.e., standalone CBBs, banks owned by a whole blood center, banks owned by a hospital, hybrid banks). We interviewed only two completely private CBBs.

We targeted transplant centers that varied with respect to the number and growth in the number of cord blood transplants conducted annually, and the ethnic and racial make-up of the populations served. We identified representatives from agencies most likely to have policies that impact cord blood collection, storage, and use. Finally, we targeted academic and private-sector researchers conducting research on potential therapeutic applications of cord blood, as well as those conducting research on cord blood itself (i.e., researchers studying the potential expansion of small CBUs).

We identified potential respondents through publicly available information, including FDA registration data, the NCBI program website, The Registry, and WMDA survey results. We also identified some respondents through professional referrals.[39, 48, 65]

We note that our sampling frame of key stakeholders does not reflect the entire population of stakeholders; therefore, our findings may not be representative. We used *purposeful* or *nonprobability sampling*, which is common in qualitative research and allows us to focus on collecting data from a limited number of respondents with specific knowledge or expertise.[66]

Protocols

We developed separate and unique interview guides for each type of respondent, focusing on each respondent group's role in the cord blood system. To develop the interview guides, we drew on findings from the literature review to form an initial set of questions for each type of interviewee. We refined the interview guides to facilitate better collection of emerging themes from early interviews. The final interview guides are available in Appendix A of this report.

Data Collection

As appropriate for semi-structured interviews, interviewers followed respondents' leads, allowing the breadth and sequence of topics to flow naturally from respondents' answers to questions. Each interview lasted from 45 to 60 minutes, was conducted by phone, and was audio-recorded (with permission). One lead interviewer and at least one notetaker conducted each interview. Most interviews were with individuals, but to accommodate respondent schedules, some were with groups of interviewees. Our notes were augmented by transcribing salient quotes from recordings and summarizing the general themes discussed in each interview.

Final Sample

In Table 3.1, we provide details on our sample of interview participants and the organizations they represent. We note that the totals in each column of participants and organizations will sum to more than the total number for each category because many participants and organizations are counted in more than one category. For instance, many of our researchers were also transplant physicians.

Table 3.1. Interview Participants and Organizations

	Number of Participants (n = 44)	Number of Organizations (n = 33)
Public CBBs	14	11
Private CBBs	9	6
Hybrid CBBs[a]	4	4
Researchers	5	5
Transplant centers	10	9
Suppliers	5	5
Other[b]	10	5

[a] Hybrid banks are listed as both private and public banks.
[b] Includes payers and government and nongovernment representatives.

Data Analysis

We created a draft of the code structure that would allow us to classify consistently concepts described by our key interviewees. We used the constant comparative method to identify novel concepts by adding codes, expanding on existing codes, or refining existing codes.[67] Two members of the research team applied the code structure to notes and transcripts from our interviews. Following Miles and Huberman,[68] the thematic analysis incorporated both themes and trends identified in our key interviews, as well as in review of documents obtained throughout the study period.[69] Our analysis generated insights into the perceptions and experiences of various stakeholders in the public cord blood system in the United States.

Cord Blood Bank Follow-Up

We contacted all the public CBBs we interviewed to answer a set of detailed follow-up questions on the costs and collection methods used at their banks. Only three banks agreed to answer the questions (21 percent), but among these three sets of responses there was significant item nonresponse. To maintain the confidentiality of the respondents, we do not report any quantitative results from this follow-up, but we provide qualitative findings where appropriate.

Quantitative Approach

Our quantitative approach included analysis of data from several different sources across multiple levels (e.g., CBU, patient, bank, and transplant). We discuss each data set and our analysis of each below. In subsequent chapters, we present a synthesis of results from various sources as appropriate for each research question.

FDA CBB Registration Data

We requested a full list of all registered active umbilical cord blood establishments operating in the United States from the FDA. These data are publicly available through the Human Cell and Tissue Establishment Registration—Public Query website,[70] and were made available to us in electronic form as of 2016.

Sample

We restricted the sample to entities operating in the United States whose product list included "umbilical cord blood stem cells."

Approach

We utilized the list of umbilical cord blood establishments paired with data from other publicly available sources (e.g., the NMDP, the WDMA) to develop a list of potential CBBs to contact for our qualitative interviews.

NMDP Data

The NMDP provided us with cord blood banking and shipment data at both the CBU level and aggregated at the bank level. We discuss each data source below.

CBU- or Patient-Level Data

We used banking data that included the TNC-count category (less than 90, 90–124, 125–149, 150–175, and more than 175) and the broad racial/ethnic category of the donor for each CBU collected (and registered on The Registry). These data covered 202,160 units added to The Registry between 2002 and 2016. The 2016 data are incomplete, so we primarily focus on 2015 as the last year of data available.

We also used cord blood shipment data that included the TNC count (continuous), the race and ethnicity of the donor and patient, whether the unit was used domestically or internationally, the broad disease category of the patient, and the year shipped for CBUs shipped between 2010 and 2016. We are missing data from October to December 2010 and from August and September 2016. From 2010 to 2016, there were 10,787 cord blood shipments both domestically and abroad, including single and multi-cord units.

Finally, we used U.S. transplant patient-level data available from January 2010 to June 2016, which included the source of HSCs, i.e., cord blood, haploidentical donor, bone marrow or other peripheral stem cells from a related donor, and from an unrelated donor; the broad disease group; the patient's age category (in ten-year increments); the patient's broad race/ethnicity category; and the year of the transplant. These data are different from the cord blood shipment data described in the previous paragraph because they do not include international shipments, and did not occur in exactly the same time frame. From 2010 to 2016, there were 52,098 transplants, including 4,958 cord blood transplants.

Approach

We used these three data sources to describe the supply and demand for cord blood, as well as how this varies by race/ethnicity and TNC count. We specifically examined trends over time in the number of units recruited and shipped by race, age, and TNC count, and we discuss this in more detail in Chapters Five and Six. We also used these data to estimate input parameters for our economic models, described in detail in Chapter Seven. For example, from these data, we can estimate the probability that a CBU with a given TNC count will be collected, banked, or used for transplant in a given year.

Bank-Level Data

In addition, the NMDP provided us with bank-level data, which included details about the number of units banked and shipped, the number of banked CBUs that were NCBI units, the number of banked CBUs in each TNC-count category, and the number for broad patient racial/ethnic categories. These data include 22 public CBBs with CBUs registered with the NMDP. We were also provided with industry-wide average financial information, including the average rate of units discarded from collection to processing and registering the units, the collection costs per collected unit costs, the processing costs per unit, and sales price. Finally, the NMDP provided bank-level cost data for four CBBs that they interviewed to provide ranges of potential costs at the bank level and estimated aggregate industry costs.

Approach

We combined the bank-level data with publicly available data on the HRSA NCBI contracts[71] (namely contract amount and year of contract) for two purposes. First, we used the bank-level data to compare NCBI banks with non-NCBI banks and to investigate the role of HRSA subsidies in determining banks' decisions on what kind of CBUs they bank. Second, combined with published literature, information from interviews, and follow-up data from three CBBs, we used the industry-wide average financial information in our economic model to determine profit maximization, which we explain in more detail in Chapter Seven.

Agency for Healthcare Research and Quality National Inpatient Sample

We used the online query tool from the Healthcare Cost and Utilization Project (HCUPnet), to examine utilization and costs of HSC transplants. We specifically examined frequencies of utilization based on hospital discharge data by patient age, payer, and year from the Agency for Healthcare Research and Quality's (AHRQ's) National Inpatient Sample (NIS)—the largest publicly available all-payer inpatient health care database in the United States.[72] We also produced aggregate statistics of length of stay, costs, and charges.

Sample

We restricted the sample to all discharges where the International Classification of Diseases, Ninth Revision, Clinical Modification (ICD-9 CM) principal procedure code was one of the following:

- 41.03: allogeneic bone marrow transplant without purging
- 41.05: allogeneic HSC transplant without purging
- 41.06: cord blood stem cell transplant
- 41.08: allogeneic HSC transplant with purging.

We focused on these procedures because they consistently have large enough sample sizes to produce descriptive statistics. *Purging* refers to myeloablative (or intense) conditioning.

Approach

Using HCUPnet, we produced descriptive statistics of average length of stay, costs, and charges, by procedure code and year. In Table 3.2 we show the sample sizes and frequency of inpatient discharges by procedure code for which we obtained descriptive statistics from HCUPnet. AHRQ has suppressed some cells (denoted as asterisks in the table). In some cases, we were able to impute the value in the cells based on other outputs (those values are italicized in the table). For example, in 2011, the total number of discharges with primary diagnosis of 41.03 is not reported. However, the number of discharges that were covered by Medicaid is reported at 288, and AHRQ reports that this is 22.09 percent of the total discharges with that primary diagnosis. Thus, we imputed the total number of discharges as 288 divided by 22.09 percent, for a total of 1,305. For most years, the frequencies are unavailable for principal procedure code 41.08, but HCUPnet does produce mean costs, charges, and length of stays for this procedure. Therefore, we report this in Chapter Six, but results should be interpreted with caution because we are not confident in the generalizability of those statistics.

Table 3.2. Frequency of Different Stem Cell Transplant Procedures and Percentage of Pediatric Procedures in the NIS, 2005–2014

Year	Allogeneic Bone Marrow, No Purging (41.03)		Allogeneic HSC, No Purging (41.05)		Cord Blood Stem Cell (41.06)		Allogeneic HSC, Purging (41.08)	
	n	% Age 1–17	n	% Age 1–17	n	% Age 1–17	n	% Age 1–17
2005	1,437	53%	3,667	*	321	49%	*	*
2006	513	*	1,928	*	*	*	*	*
2007	1,127	*	*4,175*	*	*	*	*	*
2008	1,023	*	4,933	*	*	*	*	*
2009	1,172	*	5,487	11%	666	*	*	*
2010	1,168	46%	5,149	*	693	48%	*	*
2011	*1,305*	*	4,534	*	*	*	*	*
2012	1,015	38%	4,660	9%	465	34%	*	*
2013	875	43%	4,460	9%	425	29%	*	*
2014	870	33%	5,005	9%	395	*	100	*

SOURCE: Weighted national estimates from HCUPnet NIS, 2005–2014, AHRQ, based on data collected and provided to AHRQ by individual states. Statistics based on estimates with a relative standard error (standard error / weighted estimate) of more than 0.30 or with a standard error of zero in the nationwide statistics are not reliable and have been suppressed. Beginning with the 2012 data, the NIS was redesigned to optimize national estimates. The nationwide statistics in HCUPnet for years prior to 2012 were regenerated using new trend weights to permit longitudinal analysis. The regenerated data were posted to HCUPnet on July 2, 2014. Therefore, the statistics for years prior to 2012 currently on HCUPnet will differ slightly from statistics obtained prior to July 2, 2014.

NOTE: Cells with asterisks were suppressed. Values in italics have been imputed based on other outputs, as explained in the text.

Chapter Four. Trends Affecting Public Cord Blood System Sustainability

The U.S. public cord blood system is currently in a period of financial stress, as many public CBBs are facing challenges adapting to evolving market conditions. In this chapter, we focus on understanding how key cord blood system stakeholders perceive the current challenges in a broader context of change within the entire stem cell marketplace and in the U.S. health care system. These broader systemic changes include increasing competition among both domestic and foreign CBBs; falling domestic and international demand for U.S. cord blood, in part because of a global trend toward using haploidentical sources for HSC transplantations; and shifting CBB collection and ownership structures.

The aim of this chapter is to identify and describe the most-significant trends already affecting public CBBs in the United States. To identify and understand these trends, we relied on interviews and reviewed literature and data sources, as described in Chapter Three. We limit this chapter's discussion to trends that are already established and observable, while in Chapter Eight we discuss nascent or potential future changes that could significantly impact the cord blood sector.

Leading Trends

Our analysis and key stakeholders identified several important trends affecting the U.S. public cord blood system. Many of the trends identified in our analysis are interrelated, and most of these trends are potential threats to the financial viability of public CBBs. Note that when we detail insights from hybrid CBBs, we are referring to practices on the public CBB side, unless otherwise indicated.

Below we describe each trend and provide illustrative examples, quotes, and other supporting evidence. In later chapters, we further analyze the business and policy implications of these trends for the public cord blood system.

Increased Competition Among CBBs

Most representatives from groups that we interviewed noted increased domestic and international competition among public CBBs in the United States. Two representatives of nongovernmental agencies noted that there might be "too many" public CBBs, and one researcher commented that consolidation among public CBBs "might not be a bad thing," stating

> a huge mistake was made in the beginning in terms of facilitating a
> multitude of banks. It's not a cost-efficient model. There should be banks
> of excellence.... There are a number of smaller banks we would not use
> and those banks should be allowed to fold. The transplant physicians

who have a lot of experience should be asked which banks they want to use. They're the ones who are buying the units and need to defend the cost and quality of the graft. It has not helped the field to create 30 banks. We should have less than ten and they should be a powerhouse of creating high-quality grafts around the country.

Some of this increased competition has also come from international CBBs. One expert who closely follows international cord blood sales explained that

in the beginning, our banks did have a very large market share globally…[foreign banks have] become increasingly self-sufficient. Definitely in the early days the French registry and the U.S. registries were emerging much more rapidly. There were also quite a few cord blood banks emerging around Europe. The quality of the U.S. banks was seen as a higher-quality inventory in the beginning. So some of the European banks faded away. They hadn't put a lot of effort in or they hadn't held their banks to a quality standard where they were getting a lot of requests…then, as England began its own cord blood program, especially with a specific interest in diversity, they were increasingly able to meet the demands of their diverse patients in addition to their Caucasian patients. Then we saw Asia…start forming cord blood banks and collecting inventory…there was less need to access the U.S. for cord blood units. The heyday of U.S. cord blood unit activity going overseas was probably more like four to five years ago and has started to decline.

Several researchers and transplant center representatives noted that U.S. CBUs are more expensive than foreign CBUs and may therefore be less likely to be used abroad. Data from the NMDP confirm this trend, showing that almost a quarter of U.S. CBBs' total sales used to go to foreign destinations, but this share dropped to approximately 16 percent of total sales in recent years (see Figure 4.1). U.S. cord blood sales to foreign destinations appear to have peaked in 2012 at 430 units (24.6 percent), and then gradually fell to 237 units in 2015 (14.6 percent).

In a 2011 GAO report, public banks cited competition with private banks as an important factor, with one noting that in hospitals with a more affluent population "the loss of available cord blood to private banking can exceed 20 percent."[1] Key interviewees in our study held varying opinions on the level and nature of competition between private and public CBBs. For example, one manager of a public bank stated that public banks

don't feel that they [public banks] compete with them [private banks]. We don't try to. They have a different clientele. [We are] getting units from people who aren't looking at private banking. The majority can't afford private banking. It goes into the trash if they don't donate to the public bank.

A hybrid bank representative noted that organizations such as the Cord Blood Association include both private and public banks, and that there is general cooperation between the two groups. In Chapter Eight we further discuss and analyze potentially beneficial relationships between public and private banks.

Figure 4.1. Percentage of CBUs Shipped from U.S. CBBs to Domestic and International Destinations

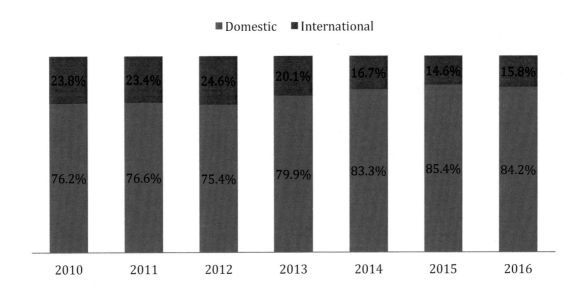

SOURCE: NMDP-provided data (see Chapter Three for details).

This competition from international CBBs is not only decreasing U.S. exports abroad, it is also decreasing U.S. cord blood sales at home. International CBBs used to supply approximately 13 percent of all CBUs used in the United States, but more recently that share has increased to approximately 24 percent, as illustrated in Figure 4.2.

Figure 4.2. Percentage of CBUs Derived from International CBBs and Sold in the United States

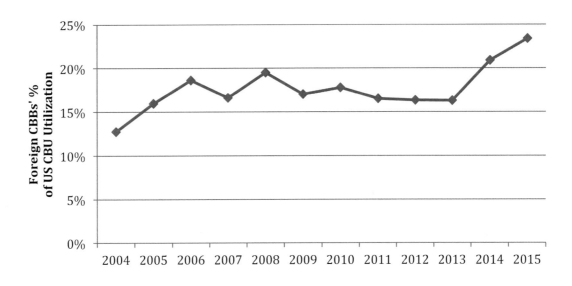

SOURCE: NMDP-provided data (see Chapter Three for details).

However, at least one public CBB representative did perceive competition with private CBBs. One public CBB leader explained, "[w]e are absolutely in competition with private CBBs because they market everywhere and are not limited in [geographic] scope."

Other key interviewees voiced concerns with some of the marketing and/or educational materials that some private CBBs disseminate to expectant parents. For instance, two respondents reported that some private banks have made unsupported statements regarding the potential uses of cord blood to encourage expectant parents to bank privately. Our own review of private CBBs' websites corroborates these statements. For instance, one private bank, ViaCord, has the following statement on its website: "Nearly 80 life-threatening diseases—from cancers to blood diseases to immune disorders—can use cord blood stem cells in treatment." The website does not point out that very few of these diseases would use autologous cord blood (as opposed to allogeneic cord blood, which would have to come from a public CBB). Further, ViaCord's website also indicates that Tay Sachs disease and osteoporosis could be treated by cord blood, even though the use of cord blood for these conditions is experimental, not scientifically proven, and not the standard of care. Two respondents reported that private banks have harmed patients by failing to maintain quality standards, thereby hurting the mission of cord blood banking overall. Both respondents—representing separate organizations—described an instance in which a hybrid CBB was using an outdated method of cell processing. After several adverse events resulting from the use of CBUs processed using this method, they stopped using this processing method on the public banking side. However, our respondents reported that this hybrid bank continued using this processing method on the private banking side, and even marketed it as a "premium method" for which it charged extra to families. One respondent said, "what [they] got was stem cells that can be lethal…there are things in the industry that aren't proper."

Decreasing Demand for Cord Blood

Of the seven public CBBs we interviewed, only one reported stable or increased cord blood sales in the past two years compared with previous years. All other public CBBs reported that their sales had fallen significantly, sometimes by nearly half, compared with prior-year sales. There was little consensus from key interviewees with regard to whether these trends would continue in the future.

A variety of secondary trends were perceived to have contributed to the decreased use of cord blood, which we discuss in more detail below. We note that many of these trends are interrelated, and it is not possible to single out an individual leading or driving trend.

Challenges of the Relatively Small Size of CBUs

CBUs generally have a smaller number of stem cells compared with other HSC transplant sources. Existing clinical guidelines recommend a TNC count of 2.5×10^7 per kg of patient weight. Given the weight of an average adult in the United States, most CBUs currently available in the national inventory have TNC counts that fall below this requirement. Using the current TNC cutoff of 0.9 billion cells used by NCBI, a CBU of this size would only be sufficient for an individual weighing 32 kg or less. Although this may be sufficient for many pediatric patients, an adult male of average weight (89 kg) in the United States would need a CBU with a TNC of at least 2.22×10^9 while an average-weight female (75 kg) would need a CBU with a TNC of at least 1.87×10^9.[73] Although a double cord blood transplant is possible, it can significantly increase costs and push the calculus of choosing an HSC source toward less-expensive alternatives, such as haploidentical transplants. NMDP data show relatively equal declines in the number of cord blood transplants using single units and double units over time.

The small size of many existing CBUs effectively shrinks the overall "usable" cord blood inventory in the United States. One representative of a hybrid CBB noted that, with regard to the existing inventory, all transplant centers are "fishing from one end of the pond" when searching for cord blood, and that the effective inventory currently useable is only about 10,000 CBUs, despite having over 200,000 units listed on The Registry.

Several respondents noted that the small size of CBUs might contribute to their higher cost, which, in turn, may lower demand for cord blood. Transplant recipients are at greater risk for infections and GVHD during the engraftment period, which is longer due to the smaller size of cord blood relative to other sources. As this transplant physician described,

> [o]nce the cord goes in, the time to recovery tends to be quite a bit slower for neutrophils and platelets than some of the other cell sources that we use. We're looking out to the fourth week before we start to see engraftment.... The patient's immune recovery is reduced compared to some of the cell sources we use. We have a lot of trouble with reactivation, serious viral infections, CMV [cytomegalovirus infection], etc. The recovery from cord blood transplant tends to be slower and sometimes more complicated than recovery from other sources.

Increasing Use of Haploidentical Transplants

The most commonly cited trend contributing to the decreased overall use of cord blood has been the rise in haploidentical transplants, particularly during the past seven years. The overwhelming consensus from public CBBs is that haploidentical HSCs are easier and cheaper to transplant with shorter engraftment periods compared with cord blood. Several public CBBs noted that the shift toward haploidentical transplants is a global trend. A representative of a nongovernmental organization observed "the turn to haploidenticals [happened] more quickly in the U.S. In 2016, we really started to notice that change in volume in Europe as well."

A manager of a large medical device manufacturer said that people at his large international corporation

> …don't expect to see changes [in these] trends. I imagine peripheral blood [haploidentical transplants] will be the preferred start for graft choice—[because they are] easy to get to.... Bone marrow requires larger volumes and multiple punctures…. Cords are hampered by the small starting material. I don't think double cord research has progressed. I don't see growth opportunities for cords at this time in the transplant setting.

Text Box 3. Haploidentical transplants

As described in Chapter Two, when performing an HSC transplant, it has traditionally been necessary for donors and recipients to have closely matched tissue types as determined by HLA proteins, which mark cells with that person's "self" profile. The body's immune cells use these markers to distinguish the body's own cells from foreign cells. Finding a high-level HLA match can pose a significant challenge for individuals with relatively rare HLA types, for which a good match can be exceedingly difficult to find. To address this problem, researchers developed a modified form of HSC transplant, known as a *haploidentical transplant*, where a healthy first-degree relative (i.e., a parent, sibling, or child) may serve as a donor. In such cases, donors can have as little as a 50-percent HLA match to the recipient.

In a haploidentical transplant, HSCs can be harvested from bone marrow or peripheral blood, and procedures are very similar to procedures for other allogeneic HSC transplants. The main innovation of the haploidentical transplant is that several days following transplant, patients receive a very high dose of Cytoxan, a chemotherapy drug that causes a sharp decline in active T-cells. Active T-cells are a major contributor to GVHD; reducing their number increases the likelihood that the transplanted cells will not be attacked as foreign, despite having up to a 50-percent mismatch between patient and donor.

At the same time, many public CBBs, as well as researchers and transplant physicians, cautioned that they had seen other trends "come and go," and that haploidentical transplants may be just the latest trend. Many respondents also expressed concern about the long-term outcomes of haploidentical transplants. One transplant physician, who is also a researcher, said

> [t]here's still the un-discussed long-term implication of a higher risk of rejection. The argument is that in the first three to four months it costs 50 percent of a cord blood transplant. [But] the high risk of relapse can cost [an additional] 50 to 60 percent. Maintenance therapy is $15,000 to $20,000 per month. That cost has not been factored in.

Although some cord blood stakeholders viewed the rise of haploidentical transplants as contributing to the decline in use of cord blood, other respondents took a more positive view of haploidentical transplantation's effects on the cord blood system, as exemplified by this transplant physician, who said

> The addition of haploidenticals has not been to the detriment of

cords, but to be an additional stem cell source so we can transplant more people and add the option of mismatched unrelated donors.

In our quantitative analysis, we did find evidence of an increase in haploidentical transplants over time (see Figure 1.1).

Due to the longer engraftment period for CBUs, defining an episode in such a relatively short period of time can disadvantage CBUs as compared with haploidenticals. As one transplant physician explained

> [i]t's expensive when you take into account not just the cost of the units, but also the clinical care…costs associated with cords…[s]uch as the fact that patients stay in the hospital longer.

A public CBB leader elaborated that

> [g]enerally, the reimbursement for [HSC] transplants is bundled. No matter the source of the cells, the bundled payment is the same. So people may be less likely to choose [cord blood] because there is less left in the bundle for other things…. [Cord blood] is probably the most expensive cell source. That's only looking at the up-front cost. The cheapest would be a related donor, then an unrelated donor, and then cord blood. Except that's for the up-front procurement costs. But if it turns out [that] the amount or severity of GVHD is less, then maybe the cheaper up-front cost is not an overall cheaper cost.

Several transplant physicians and researchers hope that if the long-term outcomes using cord blood are better compared with other alternatives, payers may reconsider existing payment models. However, one representative from a nongovernmental organization noted that long-term outcomes are not a focus of payers, and that transplant centers may not be particularly sensitive to price because HSC transplants are still very infrequent, even if they are losing money on them.

Difficulty Distinguishing Among Many Potential CBUs

Several public CBBs and transplant physicians reported that the large number of public CBBs makes it difficult for transplant centers to distinguish between high- and low-quality CBUs. Patients with common HLA types may be able to choose from a large number of CBUs. One representative of a public CBB explained that

> the [increasing] number of banks has had a number of consequences. The fracturing of the market has resulted in people offering units. The idea is to choose the best unit from wherever it may be. The decision of which is the best unit is not always clear.

Our interviewees noted that transplant centers with extensive experience performing HSC transplants and cord blood transplants use "search coordinators" who have experience identifying CBUs that are likely to result in a good outcome. However, transplant centers with little experience performing cord blood transplants are unlikely to have such a resource.

Several physicians described having preferred public CBBs because they had greater confidence in the quality of the cord blood. One transplant physician explained that there are

> published factors that predict high unit quality. So, if you happen to be a bank that has units with those characteristics, then it's highly likely based on the data that your units would be good. If your bank doesn't have units that fulfill those characteristics, it's possible your units won't be as good.

Given the complexity of selecting the most optimal unit, one public CBB representative expressed concern that less-experienced transplant centers may select a suboptimal CBU, and then, if their patient does not have a good outcome, they may be less willing to use cord blood in the future.

Delayed Cord Clamping May Also Contribute to Smaller CBUs

Delayed cord blood clamping is a recent trend whereby the obstetrician delays clamping the umbilical cord to allow continued flow of blood to the newborn for 30 to 60 seconds after birth. The practice appears to increase hemoglobin levels at birth and improve iron stores for the first few months of life, which is associated with favorable developmental effects for the infant. The American Academy of Obstetricians and Gynecologists (ACOG) and the AAP recommend delaying umbilical cord clamping by 30–60 seconds after birth.[74, 75] Delayed umbilical cord clamping was mentioned by every public CBB representative, and by several transplant centers, as posing a challenge in collecting sufficiently large CBUs. Public CBB representatives reported that they have seen varying degrees of impact from delayed umbilical cord clamping. One hybrid CBB representative noted that

> [w]e are running into the challenge of delayed cord clamping.... One hospital is advocating doing it for all deliveries. That hospital has pretty much depleted collections because after significant delayed clamping there isn't anything left in the umbilical cord to collect. One site...is looking to close in the near future. Until two years ago it was the top collection site.

In contrast, another public CBB representative reported that

> [i]t's too soon to tell. It has not had a devastating effect. All of our sites have instituted some level of delayed clamping. ACOG now recommends 60 seconds or less. The impact is marginal.

Several respondents concurred that delaying umbilical cord clamping in accordance with clinical guidelines would still leave "plenty of cord blood" for collection. However, one public CBB representative noted that some parents and practitioners were taking the practice to an extreme, with prolonged delayed clamping of the umbilical cord, which left very little, if any, cord blood to collect. Further, extreme prolonged delayed clamping can cause neonatal jaundice and hyperbilirubinemia.[76] There were concerns that this continued trend of extreme delay could significantly affect the volume of cord blood collected, but there was no overwhelming call for an end to the practice as currently recommended by medical professional societies.

Rising Cost of CBUs

Many respondents in all categories discussed the high and rising cost of cord blood as a major deterrent to its use. A transplant physician who is also a researcher lamented that "CBUs are too expensive. Given that adults frequently need a double unit [cord blood transplant]…you're looking at a graft cost of about $90,000."

The high cost of CBUs places it at a disadvantage relative to other sources of cells for HSC transplant. A transplant physician and researcher explained that

> Cord blood is in a potentially precarious position. A number of groups don't use it because of the expense. The cost of the cord is quite high. If you can do a haploidentical transplant for less and get a similar outcome, people will run to that just because of cost.

Some public CBBs also noted that the falling use of CBUs has caused them to raise their prices (or fees charged) to cover the cost of collecting those units, thereby exacerbating the rise in prices. A hybrid CBB representative commented that

> [s]ometimes the cost is prohibitive for transplant centers. It's a chicken-and-egg scenario. For CBBs to remain competitive, prices for CBUs need to decrease while usage increases.

Some government regulations may have also contributed to higher costs. The most frequently discussed government regulation was FDA licensure. Specifically, many respondents—including public CBBs, transplant physicians, and representatives of nongovernmental organizations—attributed recent increases in costs of cord blood to the costs associated with FDA licensure. A representative from a nongovernmental organization reported that

> [o]nce the application was submitted, it was a six-month process. But it was 18 months of work up to that point.... It cost a million dollars to hire a consultant, build a clean room, and expensive lab testing to validate processes. A lot of personnel were involved in a rapid fashion.

One transplant physician and researcher noted that FDA licensure places cord blood at a relative disadvantage compared with other HSC sources because

> the creation of the licensure for the cord blood banks…put a huge burden of cost on the banks.... Banks are paying a million dollars per year to keep up with regulatory demand, and none of the other [providers of] cell types have to deal with that.

Despite FDA licensure being required by law, many public CBBs have not obtained it. Some interviewees from FDA-licensed banks expressed frustration that FDA licensure had not translated into any clear advantage for licensed banks compared with unlicensed banks. For example, one public CBB leader said

> [w]e decided to pursue FDA licensure because we thought it would be enforced eventually. We thought there would be an advantage to selling our product in terms of licensure.... It was very challenging. It required more infrastructure than we had in place.... We had to borrow or get funding for those activities to get through it.... It increased our operating expenses at the bank by about $1 million/year. Money that might go into more collection goes into these regulatory standards.

Others reported concern with a lack of mechanisms to recoup the expenses of FDA licensure. For example, one public CBB leader said

> [o]ne of the challenges that we see in terms of the market [is that] it hasn't necessarily recognized how to capture that expense, hasn't recognized that licensed units should be reimbursed at a higher rate. We could charge more for the licensed units, but we're finding that...the market won't bear the higher prices.

Several transplant physicians and public CBB representatives gave the FDA credit for helping to improve CBU standardization and quality. For example, one transplant physician acknowledged some benefits of regulation, explaining that

> [i]f you look at what's happening now compared to 20 years ago, an enormous amount has been achieved—standardization, organization, accreditation. People were doing this in freezers in the back of their lab 20 to 25 years ago. It has come a long way. We need to strike a nice balance between feasibility and overregulation.

Another leader of a hybrid CBB noted that without FDA licensure, his organization would not have been well positioned to take on other profitable new businesses. He explained that

> ...having an FDA license means we can take a product through [the] FDA, and if somebody comes to us with a product like mesenchymal cells—we can do that—we can take that and get it through an IND and clinical trials—who else can do that? For example, our competitor doesn't have an FDA-licensed stem cell product like we do—they would manufacture cells and give them back to you—and what are you going to do with them? But, we can take the cells and hold them here and distribute them—like we do with cord blood.

Beyond FDA-licensure requirements, a broad array of respondents—including nongovernmental representatives, public CBB representatives, and transplant physicians—noted that more than FDA licensure, transplant centers look at accreditation status when selecting a CBU. A hybrid CBB representative reported that "...accreditation through FACT or AABB is viewed as very rigorous and at least as good as FDA [licensure]."

This was confirmed by several transplant physicians, including one who said

> [w]e pay attention to FACT accreditation. [For b]anks that have gotten their act together to submit a BLA…[it] doesn't mean that a unit from their bank is better. All of the units prior to getting a license are still good-quality units.

Finally, several respondents discussed the effect of HRSA's NCBI program, which subsidizes part of the procurement costs but are not provided every year for all contractor banks. Although HRSA sets a minimum TNC count for CBUs to be eligible for the subsidy, this cutoff is relatively low, and some respondents felt this incentivized the collection of small units. One researcher and transplant physician described the "catch-22" situation some public banks may find themselves in because they need the NCBI subsidies from HRSA for short-term cash flow, despite the fact that continuing to collect the smaller units can be harmful to banks' long-term financial sustainability.

> There are rumors that smaller units are collected from minority patients to get the HRSA money, but those units never go out the door. It also doesn't make sense to bank the smaller units because they will never be used.

This researcher and transplant physician argued that the money used to subsidize smaller CBUs with a low likelihood of usage could be better spent elsewhere.

> Doctors aren't going to take smaller units. You can bank all you want, but people aren't going to use them. People should be more comfortable making those decisions now that there are more options. Policies should not be set for the exception. We can't definitely say which option is the best, but they're all in the same ballpark. For all of the millions of dollars spent on banking things that are never used, we could do something to make a difference for transplantation, like helping to pay for transplants.

One hybrid CBB representative noted that the HRSA focus on ethnic and racially diverse units may also contribute to increasing costs.

> It's not sustainable. All the banks are losing money. They are all going to come apart. The biggest problem is that the HRSA model is wrong. HRSA is focused on banking minority units, but 70 percent of the units that get transplanted are Caucasian. From a financial standpoint, that doesn't work. They only give you half the cost of banking the units; you have to spend the other half. They set the TNC low, [and] people go after chasing small units—it's a disaster. You spend $3,000 to bank a unit from a minority patient and it's not going to get used. Statistically, it won't get used. If the government wants us to do things for the greater good, they should be paying full price for it. But from a business point of view, somebody has to pay for it.

On the other hand, this same researcher and transplant physician commented [donor ethnicity is] relevant for cord blood banking because it influences where you go to collect your cords. If you're trying to serve the African-American community, you will want a greater number of African-American cords. Financially, that doesn't help the cords much because the reason that minorities are minorities is that they're not the major group. So, the majority of people who get leukemia are Caucasian. Of course, that's changing and getting even more complicated with mixed-race [patients]. And there's, of course, the social justice aspect. All ethnicities should have a chance to find a decent donor.

CBBs Are Innovating to Meet Financial Challenges

Most public CBBs are responding to the pressures described above by adjusting their approaches to collection, diversifying into new lines of business, and exploring new ownership structures. Although no single innovative strategy has enough subscribers to constitute a clear trend, the fact that so many public CBBs are innovating in diverse ways is itself a trend that is helping to develop practices to increase efficiency and contributing to CBBs' future sustainability.

Several banks noted that to collect large and/or diverse CBUs, they have shut down collections at some hospitals and partnered with new hospitals. There was no single model of collection that was prevalent among all CBBs. Rather, the approach was tailored to the hospitals available and the experience of the CBB. One leader of a public CBB described his organization's approach:

> To move into a hospital, we look at the birth rate and the ethnicity of the births, [a]nd see if we think that will be a good place to go through the trouble of setting up collections. Then we need to have local champions. In order to shut down a collection, it's when all those things don't work.

At least two other public CBBs have diversified their inventory of CBUs by establishing partnerships with geographically distant collection hospitals. This is a break from traditional practices because most CBBs collect from hospitals that are in the same state or region of the country. For example, one public CBB representative explained that his organization ships units across the Pacific Ocean to a partner CBB that processes and banks the units.

> [W]e collect...97-percent minority units...25 percent of the units we send get banked...not bad considering they have to fly across the ocean.

A manager of another hybrid CBB shared that his organization used to collect in-state, but now collects from two neighboring states that tend to yield CBUs with higher cell counts.

Other public CBBs have shifted expensive, labor-intensive procedures, such as the detailed maternal questionnaire, until after the unit is determined to be of sufficient size.

> [We are] trying an all-collect model…everyone is asked and consented and then [we only] go to moms whose units were big enough and get full consent and ask them to give a [blood] sample [and] full questionnaire.

Another public CBB noted that they had a policy of having anything that was collected come to their lab for processing.

> Our process is that we have all of the cord blood units that are collected sent to us. We don't do triage in the hospital. [Ours is] a high-collection–high-output model. Shipping is done by big daily batches. There's no shipping cost reduction if we send less units. We anticipate someday being able to use all of them. We wanted them to all come here, which is unusual for the industry.

One hybrid CBB has a collection strategy that focuses on utilization rates. As the CBB manager explained,

> [w]e look at the utilization rate of different groups of cords. What is the utilization rate, how many units do you have, and how much is a unit worth? You don't want to spend $3,000 for something that, after you get in the bank, is worth $300. You are losing money in that case. You've got to be banking ones that have a higher utilization rate.

Public CBBs have also attempted to diversify sources of revenue by expanding the services and products they provide. Public CBBs that are becoming hybrid banks by expanding into private cord blood banking are the most obvious example of this trend. Several CBBs mentioned that hybrid banks are attractive primarily because the private side can compensate for the financial losses incurred on the public side. For example, one manager of a hybrid CBB stated that

> [i]t's fair to say we'd never make a profit on the public side—it is a loss every year—we absorb that and we recognize that for what it is…. This was never profit-driven and [we] never sought to make money off of this [public banking]. The draw to this was to give back because I don't think anyone believes you can make money with public banking.

Another manager of a different hybrid bank stated

> [w]e started as a hybrid bank to get financial support for the public bank…. Public banking isn't profitable. Because of the private banking I'm able to generate revenue to cover [public-banking] expenses or losses.

Among public CBBs that are not hybrids, some are considering the option. One manager of a public CBB stated

> [w]e have reached out to the community to look into setting up a private banking program to subsidize the public banking program.

Several public CBBs also noted that they have adjusted their business models to sell services to private CBBs. For instance, some public CBBs provide processing and storage services for private CBBs, as described by a representative of a hybrid bank that had

41

moved away from marketing their own private bank toward providing processing and storage for other private banks.

> [Business with private banks] has allowed us to generate a small revenue at the end of the year. Even with the expenses, public banking isn't profitable. Because of the private banking, I'm able to generate revenue to cover expenses or losses.

Some public CBBs have also diversified into services and products not related to cord blood banking. One hybrid CBB representative we interviewed has expanded into HLA testing, mesenchymal stem cells (MSCs), diabetic wound healing, and chimeric antigen receptor (CAR) T-cell work in additional to stem cell processing and cord blood banking. A manager there explained

> I don't think you can just run a CBB by itself today—it doesn't make sense to me. Cord blood banking needs to be part of a stem cell enterprise that's bigger—it doesn't make sense on its own—it's too esoteric on its own…. If you are only a CBB, it doesn't pay off.

CBBs have also explored a variety of ownership structures that may bolster their sustainability. Some public CBBs are strategically located within a larger entity, such as a blood center or a biotechnology company. Several representatives of public CBBs owned by a blood bank stated that their cord blood programs benefit from using the couriers, labs, and hospital connections of their whole blood programs. One representative of a hybrid CBB noted that

> [o]ur bank shares a footprint with a blood center. The biggest benefit is the logistical part of moving units from collection hubs to our processing center. It saves us from hiring additional overnight couriers. We also rely upon the lab functions of the blood center.

Other public CBBs are owned by hospitals, and this appears to confer some advantages. A leader of one of these CBBs explained that

> [w]e can also do the transplants here because we have the patients. We have a lot of advantages over competitors…[we] can bring in the top talent. But, if you are a cord blood bank [that] doesn't do transplants…is that going to work, or are you going to focus on banking? [C]ord blood banking needs to be part of a stem cell enterprise that's bigger.

Summary

Our interviews indicate that most public CBBs are facing increasing competition to provide CBUs in the face of decreasing demand. At the same time, CBBs are continuing to innovate to meet these challenges. The changing competitive landscape includes competition between public CBBs, between domestic and foreign CBBs, and possibly between public and private CBBs. There is also substitutability across HSC sources.

The decreasing demand and increasing competitive environment was perceived to have resulted from several factors. First, many respondents attributed the decrease in the use of cord blood to the corresponding increase in haploidentical transplants, which are usually less expensive. CBUs are also relatively smaller in size compared with other HSC sources, resulting in a longer engraftment period and an accompanying risk for infections. Delayed umbilical cord clamping can also result in decreased size of collected CBUs. Additionally, inexperienced transplant centers may find it difficult to select the most appropriate CBU among many potential matches. Finally, some respondents perceived that some federal regulations—such as FDA licensure requirements and the HRSA NCBI program—have contributed to the rising cost of CBUs.

Despite these complex challenges, we found that CBBs continue to innovate to meet the financial challenges they face. This includes developing and implementing innovative collection strategies, diversifying their sources of revenue, and exploring new ownership and/or organizational structures that may help them to remain financially viable into the future. There are no clear indications about whether these trends have stabilized or whether they will continue. Later chapters will explore the potential implications if some of these trends continue, or if other developments were to disrupt the U.S. cord blood system, and will also examine the economic and financial effects of current policies.

Chapter Five. Trends in Public Cord Blood Banking and Shipping

In this chapter, we highlight several of the unique properties of cord blood that have a significant effect on how the cord blood market functions, including how market participants make decisions regarding investments in inventory, pricing, subsidies, and organizational structures. We briefly highlight some unusual market characteristics present in the cord blood system, organized by the cord blood physical characteristics responsible for these market characteristics. Finally, we used data from the NMDP to show trends in the banking and shipping of cord blood over time, as well as by key cord blood characteristics (see Chapter Three for a full description of this data source).

Uniqueness of Cord Blood

Cord Blood Saves Lives and Consists of Living Human Cells

The fact that cord blood transplantation is a life-saving intervention and that cord blood is itself alive significantly affect several aspects of the cord blood market. Parents of newborns make the altruistic decision to donate neonatal tissue at the time of birth, and often hospital staff donate their labor and facilities to collect cord blood on behalf of CBBs. These are the two most obvious examples of altruism outweighing any profit motive among market participants, but this altruism is also evident among CBB managers and government officials, who often attribute their policies and business decisions to goals other than financial profit, including the goal of saving lives.

Furthermore, because cord blood consists of living human cells, market participants sometimes refrain from valuing it the way that they might value other products, such as rice. For example, supermarkets do not hesitate to differentiate the prices of different bags of rice according to weight, type, quality, supply, and demand. However, CBBs refrain from doing so, typically pricing all their CBUs equally despite significant variation in demand for CBUs of different sizes and HLA types. Because the market for rice is priced flexibly, farmers, processors, and sellers are more likely to feel price incentives to meet the needs of the marketplace. However, CBBs often bank units that are not in the highest demand, in part because cord blood's inflexible pricing gives them less financial incentive to cater to the needs of the market.

Additionally, because the cord blood market consists of real people whose lives depend on a life-saving transplant, issues of equity and fairness sometimes outweigh profit incentives. People involved in subsidizing and banking units have sometimes proven willing to bank units with a lower probability of use to serve minority populations who are statistically less likely to get a cord blood transplant.

Cord Blood Can Be Frozen for Decades

Unlike many products, cord blood has a long shelf life—20 years or more—which carries many economic implications. Unlike perishable products that cannot be frozen, cord blood can be shipped internationally. In practice, U.S. hospitals often purchase cord blood from foreign countries, and vice versa, making the U.S. market impossible to analyze without considering foreign supply and demand.

Also, because decades may pass between the time of collection and the time of sale, public banking is a capital-intensive enterprise. As described below, CBBs incur most of their procurement costs during the first week after collection, while most of their revenue is realized years—even decades—later. This is the opposite of the "just-in-time" model that made Japanese car manufacturers so profitable, and may be a significant cause of CBBs' lack of profitability. This also contrasts with the market characteristics of haploidentical HSC transplantation, which always incurs the majority of costs close to its time of use.

Cord blood's long shelf life may provide some investment value, however, in addition to its immediate value. Currently, most cord blood sold in the United States is used for transplantation in patients requiring new bone marrow, and, presumably, hospitals and payers will only be willing to pay for this portion of the cord blood's value. However, if future research discovers new medical applications for cord blood, already-banked CBUs may last long enough to be sold. This investment value is difficult to quantify, but research indicates that expansion technologies and new medical applications for cord blood are promising enough to tempt at least some investors to bet on cord blood's future.

Despite the extreme diversity of human HLA types, cord blood's long shelf life makes it feasible for U.S. and global inventories to someday fully or partially match to almost every possible patient. Demand for cord blood may increase as the inventory becomes more complete and cord blood provides a closer match to an increasing number of patients.

Cord Blood and Its Consumers Are Extremely Genetically Diverse

As noted earlier, the cord blood system must collect significantly more units than would likely be used at any one time to ensure that a given patient will have a match. This also means that the probability that any specific unit will be used in a given year will be low. This leads to an unusual market situation, whereby thousands of units of product have been collected but have not been used. These unused CBUs are not considered "wasted," in that they could potentially be used if a matching patient comes along. However, many future patients who will need these CBUs have not yet been born or have not yet become sick, making the exact demand for HLA types unknowable. The effect of the difference between collection and use has significant economic implications at the bank level, which we will discuss more in subsequent chapters.

Supply and Demand of Cord Blood Units

As noted in the introduction, the overall use of HSCs has increased over time, from slightly more than 7,000 transplants in 2010 to almost 9,000 in 2015 (see Figure 1.1). After the first year of NCBI funding for contractor banks (FY 2006), the inventory of CBUs banked and registered has increased, with more than 200,000 CBUs currently listed.[77] Despite some year-to-year fluctuations in the number of units added to the national cord blood inventory, the number added has declined since the last cohort of banks was added to the program in 2010 (see Figure 5.1). The percentage of HSC transplants that used cord blood as the HSC source has declined from about 12 percent to 7 percent.

In this report, we refer to units added to the The Registry as *banked* or *stored*, and we use these two descriptive terms interchangeably. We refer to units that have been shipped or released for use in a transplant as *shipped CBUs*. The number of CBUs shipped each year reflects the annual demand for cord blood that is met by the current market. There may also be patients who would prefer cord blood, but for whom high-quality units are not available. The difference between the cumulative number of banked units and units shipped over a certain period represents the supply of cord blood or units potentially available for transplantation. In the next sections, we present trends in both banked and shipped units, often stratified by key characteristics.

CBUs' TNC Counts

As described in Chapter Two, the TNC count is an important aspect physicians consider when selecting a CBU for transplant, because it is highly correlated with transplant success. Although the average value of TNC count for transplanted units has remained fairly constant between 2010 and 2016—with around 75 percent of all units shipped for transplant having a TNC count of 1.50×10^9 or above—the average TNC count of the CBUs added to The Registry each year has changed over time, as presented in Figure 5.1. Between 2002 and 2004, nearly 50 percent of all units added to The Registry had a TNC count of less than 0.90×10^9, a third had a TNC count between 0.90 and 1.24×10^9, and less than 20 percent combined had a TNC count larger than 1.25×10^9. Overall, banks have increased the average size of the units they are collecting over time.

Nonetheless, a large percentage of the banked units in the United States still have lower TNC counts, and the TNC composition of the banked units does not yet match that of the units shipped for transplant. Figure 5.2 describes the TNC composition of all CBUs stored and shipped for transplant between 2010 and 2016. About 70 percent of all units added to The Registry during this period had a TNC count below 1.50×10^9 (green, purple, and light blue sections in the pie chart on the left in Figure 5.2), whereas only a quarter of all shipped units during this period had a TNC count above 1.50×10^9 (red and dark blue sections).

Figure 5.1. Annual Number of CBUs Banked by U.S. CBBs, by TNC Count

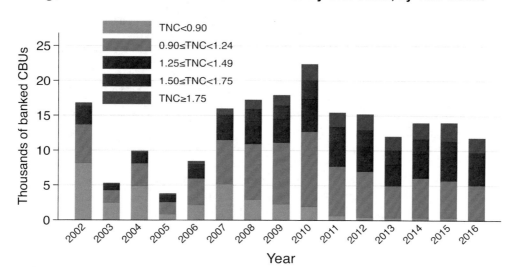

NOTE: RAND authors' calculations using NMDP data (see Chapter Three for more details on this data source). TNC count is expressed in 10^9 units.

Figure 5.2. Share of CBUs Banked and Shipped by U.S. CBBs, by TNC Count

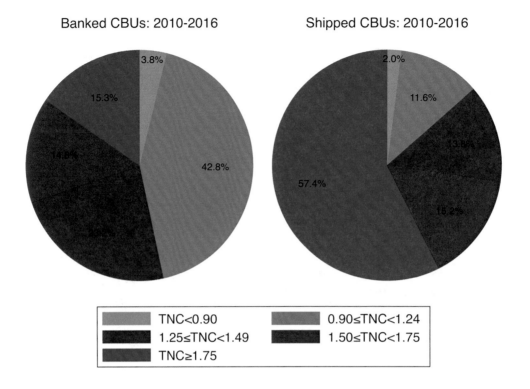

NOTE: RAND authors' calculations using NMDP data from 2002 to 2016 (see Chapter Three for more details on this data source). The term *banked CBUs* refers to CBUs collected, and *shipped CBUs* refers to CBUs released for transplant. TNC count is expressed in 10^9 units.

Donor and Patient Race/Ethnicity

Figure 5.3 shows the share of newly banked CBUs each year between 2002 and 2016 by the race/ethnicity of the donor. Since the start of the NCBI program, the share of newly banked CBUs from Caucasian donors has decreased from 65 percent (in 2006) to about 42 percent in 2015. From 2006 to 2015, the share of newly banked African-American and Hispanic CBUs increased from 8 percent to 12 percent and 14 percent to 25 percent, respectively. Since 2006, banks have added around 2,000 new units from non-Caucasians per year. A similar pattern exists for units shipped.

Figure 5.3. Percentage of Newly Banked CBUs Annually in the United States, by Race/Ethnicity

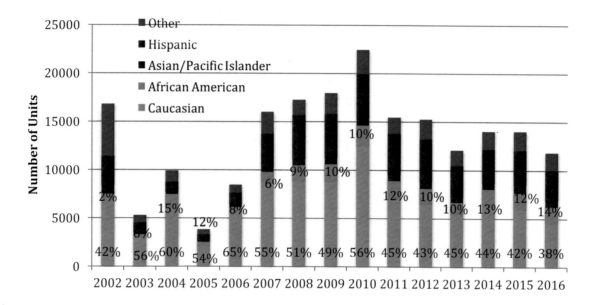

NOTE: RAND authors' calculations using NMDP data (see Chapter Three for more details on this data source). The top percentage in each column reflects the percentage of CBUs added to the inventory in a given year that were from African-American donors and the bottom percentage in the column reflects the percentage of CBUs added in a given year that were from Caucasian donors. *Other* refers to other ethnic or racial groups, to those who declined to reveal their race or ethnicity, or to those for whom race or ethnicity is unknown. As noted in Chapter Three, 2016 data is missing for two months. Because these charts show percentages, partial 2016 data is still comparable with the data for other years.

Figure 5.4 shows that, on average, the TNC count among banked CBUs does not vary substantially across race or ethnicity, but Caucasians tend to have more of the higher TNC-count units available (i.e., a smaller percentage of units donated by Caucasians have TNC counts of less than 1.25 billion). Ideally, we would like to describe the distribution of TNC-count value by race or ethnicity for CBUs collected as well as CBUs banked. However, due to data constraints, we are only able to describe distribution of units by TNC count for CBUs that are already banked and registered with the NMDP.

Despite having a larger percentage of lower–TNC count units in inventory among minority donors, the median TNC count of units used in transplantation is actually quite similar across racial and ethnic groups (see the horizontal line within each box in Figure 5.5). The median TNC value for Caucasians is 1.94×10^9, 1.81×10^9 for Hispanics, 1.75×10^9 for African-Americans, and 1.70×10^9 for Asians or Pacific Islanders. The median TNC count for Caucasians is statistically significantly different from the median TNC counts of other races or ethnicities; however, the other race/ethnicity medians are not statistically significantly different from each other.

Figure 5.4. Share of Banked CBUs Within Racial/Ethnic Categories, by TNC Count, 2002–2016

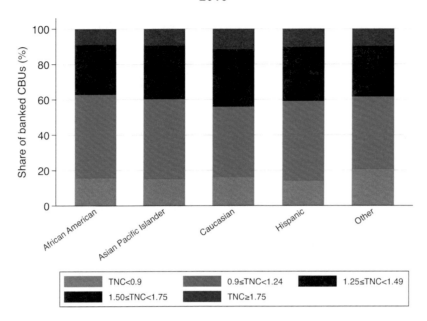

NOTE: RAND authors' calculations using NMDP data from 2002 to 2016 (see Chapter Three for more details on this data source). *Other* refers to other ethnic or racial groups, to those who declined to reveal their race or ethnicity, or to those for whom race or ethnicity is unknown. TNC count is expressed in 10^9 units.

Figure 5.5. TNC-Count Medians and Quartiles of Shipped CBUs, by Donor Race/Ethnicity

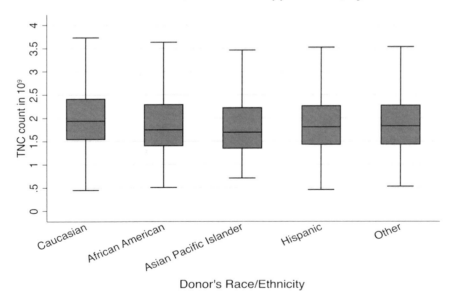

Donor's Race/Ethnicity

NOTE: RAND authors' calculations using NMDP shipment data from 2010 to 2016 (see Chapter Three for more details on this data source). Shipments include domestic and international shipments by U.S. CBBs. *Other* refers to other ethnic or racial groups, to those who declined to reveal their race or ethnicity, or for whom race or ethnicity is unknown. The ends of the "whiskers" show the first quartile (bottom) and the third quartile (top) of the TNC values for shipped CBUs. The horizontal bars in the center of the boxes represent the median TNC values.

The percentage of cord blood transplant patients who use units with TNC counts between 0.90×10^9 and 1.10×10^9 is relatively low, especially in more-recent years (see Table 5.1). Over the full study period, about 7 percent of racial/ethnic minority cord blood transplant patients utilized a low–TNC count unit. This percentage has declined over time, with only about 2–5 percent of minority patients using such units in 2016. Unfortunately, we do not have the patients' ages in these shipment-level data and therefore cannot determine whether these are primarily pediatric patients, in which case smaller units may be clinically appropriate.

Table 5.1. Percentage of Transplants Using Low–TNC Count CBUs, by Race/Ethnicity and Year

Race/Ethnicity	2010 (%)	2011 (%)	2012 (%)	2013 (%)	2014 (%)	2015 (%)	2016 (%)	Total (%)
African-American	9	7	10	4	10	7	2	7
Asian or Pacific Islander	10	6	8	7	8	5	4	7
Caucasian	7	4	5	4	4	4	3	4
Hispanic	8	6	6	5	10	7	5	7
Other	8	6	6	6	9	8	5	7

SOURCE: RAND authors' calculations using NMDP shipment data from 2010 to 2016 (see Chapter Three for more details on this data source)
NOTE: Percentages represent the number of transplants using a low–TNC count unit (between 0.9 and 1.1 billion) within a given year and racial/ethnic category, divided by the total number of transplants for that group in that year. We have excluded cord blood transplants from 2010 to 2016 with CBUs with TNC counts of less than 0.9×10^9, because those would have been with non-NCBI units. This results in dropping 230 transplants. Shipments include both domestic and international shipments by U.S. CBBs. *Other* refers to other ethnic or racial groups, to those who declined to reveal their race or ethnicity, or for whom race or ethnicity is unknown.

Adult and Pediatric Patients

A larger percentage of the Caucasian CBUs are used for adult patients, whereas pediatric use is as common or more common among African-American and Hispanic patients (see Figure 5.6).

Figure 5.6. Number of CBUs Shipped by U.S. CBBs for Pediatric and Adult Patients, by Race/Ethnicity

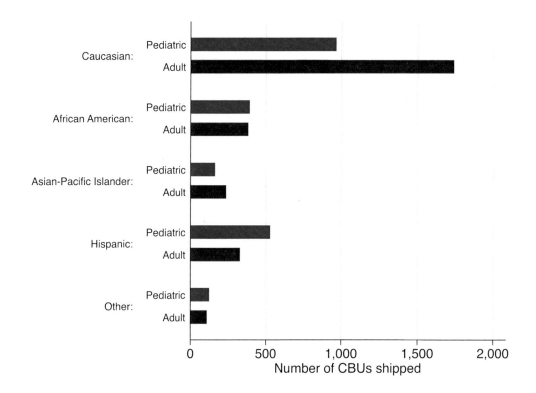

SOURCE: RAND authors' calculations using NMDP shipment data from 2010 to 2016 (see Chapter Three for more details on this data source).
NOTE: *Pediatric* refers to patients younger than 20 years old and *adult* refers to patients that are 20 years old and over. *Other* refers to other ethnic or racial groups, to those who declined to reveal their race or ethnicity, or to those for whom race or ethnicity is unknown. *CBUs shipped* refers to those shipped both domestically and internationally.

Summary

In this chapter, we discussed the unique attributes of cord blood that likely influence the economic interactions in the market. Namely, cord blood saves lives, and quantifying the value of such a treatment is complicated; cord blood can be stored for a long time; the inventory of cord blood must be significantly larger than the units needed at any given time to meet the demands of genetic diversity; and cord blood competes somewhat with other HSC sources, but in some cases it is the only option for patients (i.e., when there is no other match or they do not have time to wait).

We presented the trends showing the decline in the demand for cord blood, the growth in the national inventory, and how this varies by TNC count and racial/ethnic diversity. Nearly half of the national inventory comprised CBUs with TNC counts of less than 1.25 billion, which is problematic because these units are very unlikely to be used unless cord blood expansion technologies take off (see Chapter Eight). Although the diversity of the units has increased over time, it is unclear whether that translates into more-equitable access.

Chapter Six. Economics of Cord Blood

In this chapter, we describe the economic relationships and transactions between participants in the cord blood sector, which includes public CBBs, transplant centers and physicians, patients needing HSC transplants, and the NMDP. There are multiple economic relationships governing transactions related to cord blood, with products flowing from CBBs to hospitals (or providers), public and private health care payers providing reimbursement to providers for cord blood transplants and related care, government organizations subsidizing the collection and sale of CBUs, and patients paying insurance premiums (and cost-sharing) to payers in return for coverage of care.

We focus first on banks, presenting a description of costs related to processing and banking the CBUs and the revenue sources for CBBs. We then present details on the costs and benefits of treatment from a patient's perspective, including information on payment for and utilization of CBUs as well as highlights of the state of the evidence on clinical effectiveness of HSC transplants.

For these analyses, we relied on several sources of data, including semi-structured interviews with CBBs, their suppliers, hospitals, researchers, payers, and government regulators who have provided context and insight into the costs and benefits of cord blood. Additionally, we used NMDP data on recruitment and shipments of CBUs over time and HCUP data on inpatient stays. Finally, we supplemented these sources of information with estimates from published literature. We described our methods in more detail in Chapter Three.

Bank Costs and Revenues from Cord Blood Banking

Figure 6.1 presents an overview of the key steps that a unit goes through before being stored and later released for transplant and the costs associated with collection, testing, processing, storage, and release of the CBUs (see Chapter Two for a detailed overview of each of the steps). Although this may not be exhaustive and varies by individual CBB, this figure provides a summary of typical steps, discard rates, and costs incurred. *Discard rates* include all CBUs not used for transplant, but it does not necessarily mean that the units were not used in research or for other purposes.

Variable and Fixed Costs of Cord Blood Banking

Public CBBs incur both variable and fixed costs. *Variable costs* include costs of collection, testing, processing, storing, and distributing the unit. *Fixed costs* include obtaining FDA licensure and overhead costs, such as rent.

In Table 6.1, we present the average or range of the variable costs for each stage of the banking process for public banks, based on our interviews, bank-level data from the NMDP, and other published studies.[78–82] Collection costs include costs of recruiting donors, collection kit supplies, and labor costs. These costs may vary based on the recruitment efforts conducted, as well as whether the bank uses volunteer CBU collectors (which is most common), or whether it employs its own CBU collectors. After CBUs are collected and have arrived at the CBBs, they undergo a variety of tests, including tests for volume and weight, quality, and microbacterial contamination.

Figure 6.1. Overview of Variable Costs in a Public CBB

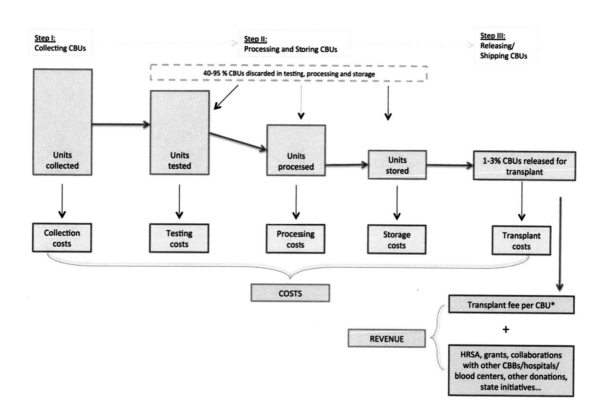

NOTES: Purple boxes denote the number of units at each stage of the CBB supply chain. Orange boxes denote the costs incurred by CBBs at each stage. Standard economic theory assumes that CBBs optimize based on costs and revenues. * Transplant fees are paid directly to CBBs from the NMDP in most cases: Transplant centers then pay the NMDP.

There are also significant costs at the processing stage, including separation of the CBU components and HLA-typing to prepare the units for storage. The cost of annual storage for a given unit is relatively small. Once CBUs are chosen for release, a small share of them may be discarded due to issues related to thawing or transportation. However, based on our interviews with CBBs and transplant physicians, this is a rare event. Distribution costs do not include the costs transplant centers incur for washing, thawing, and preparing units for transplant.

Table 6.1. Typical Variable Costs per CBU

Stage	Variable Costs per CBU	Discard Rate	Percentage of Total Variable Costs per Banked CBU
Collection/recruitment	$200	N/A	12–17%
Testing		5–65%	39–60%
Maternal infectious disease	$150		
Measuring TNC count	$100		
CD34 markers	$150–200		
Microbacterial contamination	$75		
Other	$200–250		
Total	*$675–775*		
Processing		5–25%	20–48%
Separation	$250–450		
HLA-typing	$65–125		
Total	*$315–575*		
Storage per year	$10–50	N/A	N/A
Transplant/release costs	$500–1,500	N/A	N/A
Total	$1,700–3,100		

SOURCES: Interviews and data sources cited in Todd; Wagner et al.; Jones et al.; Lauber et al.; and Lecchi et al.[78–82]
NOTE: N/A = not applicable.

Prior to the collection of CBUs, public CBBs must first register with the FDA and—since October 2011—CBBs are technically required to apply for an FDA license. The costs banks typically incur to obtain the FDA license are not publicly available. However, all respondents we interviewed agreed that the FDA licensure process is lengthy and expensive. According to these interviews, CBBs took between one and seven years to get licensed.

Average annual overhead costs—which consist of equipment costs, maintenance, rent, utilities, office supplies, and other related expenses—total from $1.2 million to $4.5 million, depending on the size and setup of the CBB.

Revenue

Public CBBs' revenues mostly depend on the fees charged to hospitals when a CBU is sold. CBBs do not typically charge different fees based on unit size, quality, or individual processing and storage costs, although costs may vary across these dimensions. For example, obtaining higher–TNC count units costs more than does obtaining lower–TNC count units, because, on average, many units must be collected to acquire a higher–TNC count unit. By contrast, the probability of obtaining a lower–TNC count unit is much higher, so it is easier and less costly to obtain those. For example, as we show in Chapter Seven, the probability that any randomly collected CBU has a TNC count of 0.9 billion or higher is about 60 percent, whereas the probability that a randomly collected unit has a TNC count of 1.5 billion or more is only about 27 percent. On the other hand, lower–TNC count units are likely to require longer storage periods, implying greater average storage costs as TNC count declines.

Because higher–TNC count units tend to be in higher demand (clinical evidence suggests better outcomes from larger units), we might expect CBBs to charge a higher price for higher–TNC count units—but we do not observe such behavior in the actual market for CBUs. In the United States, fees charged per shipped CBU vary from around $29,000 to $45,000. Based on data from our interviews, the average price per shipped CBUs is around $36,200.[79]

HRSA NCBI Contracts: Subsidies

Since 2005, the Stem Cell Therapeutic and Research Act made available $15–23 million per year for cord blood–related programs.[45] NCBI is part of this act and allows for subsidies for banked units listed on The Registry with TNC counts higher than 0.9×10^9. Subsidies per banked unit vary across public CBBs, but our estimate of the HRSA subsidy per banked CBU is approximately $1,200. Around 60 percent of all banked CBUs on The Registry are NCBI CBUs. Chapter Two describes these subsidy programs in more detail.

Other Donations and Research Grants

CBBs derive a small income stream from other federal support, charity or philanthropic donations, and research grants. For example, at the Michigan Blood CBB, contributions and grants made up only about 1 percent of all revenue in 2015 while the vast majority of revenue originated from blood products and testing.[84] Many local programs or facilities help public banks to receive donations as well. There are several state-level initiatives, such as donations in the form of a $2 fee per birth certificate in California, or granting income tax refunds toward a statewide cord blood banking program, available in Arkansas.[85–87] Several banks have actively used fundraising events to increase their income stream. For instance, GenCure, a parent organization of the Texas Cord Blood Bank, has actively used fundraising events to bridge the gap not covered by operational revenue, reporting contributions of $651,000 in 2015, out of which $96,000 were related to cord blood activities.[84] In another example, the Cleveland Foundation has awarded over $150,000 to the Cleveland Cord Blood Center, which reported combined philanthropic funding of $12.4 million between 2007 and 2014.[56, 88]

Costs and Clinical Benefits from Treatment

Above, we discussed details of the costs to CBBs of collecting, testing, processing, and storing CBUs as they relate to the price CBBs charge hospitals for CBUs. In this section, we discuss how payment for HSC transplants works, including estimates of the treatment costs of HSC transplants, drivers of costs, and current issues with costs. Because transplant physicians typically begin a search with the NMDP for *any* HSC source (cord blood, bone marrow, or other peripheral stem cell), we present much of this discussion and analysis stratifying by source where possible. As shown in Figure 2.1 and discussed in Chapter Two, the NMDP facilitates the transaction between hospitals and CBBs. Thus, payment for transplants flows from payers to hospitals and from hospitals to the NMDP for CBUs when they are used. We also consider possible changes in payment methodologies and how that could affect the market for cord blood.

Factors Affecting Treatment Costs

Differences in treatment costs to hospitals due to graft type or source of HSCs have been previously noted, with allogeneic sources and CBUs resulting in higher collection costs.[89] Although the NMDP will charge hospitals differently based on the HSC source—which is directly a function of collection costs—several studies have noted that a large share of these differences can be explained by patient factors or conditioning and not by graft types alone.[90–92] If certain conditions are treated systematically using one particular graft source, it may be difficult to disentangle how much of the cost difference is driven by differences in patient characteristics and the actual costs of treatment. For example, if higher-risk patients tend to be less likely to find a bone marrow match (i.e., they do not have time to wait to find a match), and therefore are more likely to obtain a cord blood transplant, cord blood transplants may appear costlier overall, simply because the individuals receiving those transplants tend to be sicker and require more care. We also show below that the HSC transplant costs hospitals pay that are attributable to the HSC source are a small percentage of the overall costs.

HSC transplants can occur in both outpatient and inpatient settings, but the vast majority of cord blood transplants occurs in inpatient settings. Because engraftment after transplant takes 25 to 42 days,[43] on average, these patients typically need to be isolated in an inpatient setting to prevent infection and to increase the chance of a successful engraftment. Other types of HSC transplants occur more frequently in outpatient settings, which can decrease the cost of the treatment in the short term, but this may be at least partly because higher-risk (and hence more-costly) patients tend to have transplants in inpatient settings.[93]

A related cost factor is the conditioning regimen a patient undergoes, which can vary considerably in terms of intensity and length of time. *Conditioning* is the process of preparing a recipient's bone marrow to receive an HSC transplant. How the conditioning affects the success of the transplant can ultimately affect the costs and the length of the hospital stay. Several studies have shown reduced costs with lower-intensity conditioning compared with myeloablative (more-intense) conditioning, but one study following individuals one year after transplant found no significant difference in costs.[91, 94–96]

In our investigation of HCUP inpatient discharge data for 2014 (the most-recent year for which data were available), we found significant variation across graft types, with autologous bone marrow (41.01) and other peripheral stem cells (41.04) being much less expensive during the first year and resulting in shorter lengths of stay than transplants from allogeneic sources (see Table 6.2). The two autologous transplants had inpatient costs, on average, from $56,125 to $68,382 relative to $129,514 to $262,972 for the allogeneic transplants. We note that these averages have been unadjusted for disease, setting, conditioning, or other factors that might explain differences in costs and are only reflective of inpatient stays (see Chapter Three for more details). Costs are also derived from hospital-wide cost-to-charge ratios from reports hospitals submit to the Centers for Medicare and Medicaid Services (CMS); more generally, acquisition costs reported in claims data may not reflect true transplant costs.[97] Among all allogeneic transplant procedures in inpatient settings (41.03, 41.05, 41.06, and 41.08), cord blood resulted in the longest length of stay at 51 days compared with 31 to 38 days for bone marrow or other peripheral stem cells. Not surprisingly, inpatient stay costs for cord blood transplants were significantly higher than for other types of HSC transplants at $262,972, but we note that these charges in the HCUP data only include amounts billed by hospitals. For example, other transplant patients may have additional outpatient visits, home care, and costs from relapse or GVHD that are not captured here. The medical costs of the bone marrow or peripheral stem cell donor collection are also not included here and typically are not included in cost-effectiveness analyses. These analyses also do not account for the amount of time it typically takes to obtain a bone marrow or peripheral stem donation, which, according to our interviews, can take a couple of months, on average. In a more-recent study that examined costs over a longer time period, these differences across types of transplant become less significant.[98] We also point out that the type of treatment chosen for a given patient likely depends on patient-level characteristics that may also be cost drivers, such as disease severity, comorbidities, and age.

Table 6.2. Average Length of Stay, Charges, and Costs for Inpatient HSC Transplants, 2014

ICD-9 Procedure Codes	Frequency	Average Length of Stay (days)	Average Hospital Charges	Average Hospital Costs
41.01 Autologous bone marrow transplant without purging	385	19.6 (1.01)	$173,673 ($23,521)	$68,382 ($8,325)
41.03 Allogeneic bone marrow transplant without purging	860	37.5 (2.49)	$484,745 ($45,026)	$159,005 ($13,255)
41.04 Autologous HSC transplant without purging	7,865	18.5 (0.41)	$196,532 ($8,403)	$56,125 ($2,407)
41.05 Allogeneic HSC transplant without purging	5,005	30.6 (1.19)	$419,254 ($19,032)	$129,514 ($7,185)
41.06 Cord blood stem cell transplant	395	51.2 (6.14)	$830,870 ($99,279)	$262,972 ($34,384)
41.08 Allogeneic HSC transplant with purging	100	33.5 (1.94)	$571,112 ($96,213)	$165,524 ($26,299)

SOURCE: HCUPnet 2014 National Inpatient Sample (see Chapter Three).
NOTES: Standard errors in parentheses. Total charges were converted to costs using cost-to-charge ratios based on hospital accounting reports from CMS. In general, costs are less than charges. For each hospital, a hospital-wide cost-to-charge ratio is used because detailed charges are not available across all HCUP states.

Evidence on the relationship between patient characteristics and treatment cost is less clear. As expected, patients at more-advanced stages of disease tend to have higher treatment costs, but whether this is due to some aspect of the cord blood transplant or simply due to the fact that sicker patients may require more post-transplant care is unclear.[92, 99, 100] Among pediatric patients, one study found that older children (above age ten) had higher costs, but overall, pediatric patients also tend to be more costly.[100, 101] Costs also varied by the condition for which the patient was being treated, but all these factors are likely to affect decisions about conditioning, graft type, and HSC source, as well as health care setting. Moreover, HSC transplants in inpatient settings will typically be reimbursed based on the episode, which may include a risk adjustment for patient-level factors.

Current Payment Policies

As with other parts of health care, payment rates and rules vary by payer and health care setting. Cord blood transplants typically occur in inpatient settings, but other types of HSC transplants occur more frequently in outpatient settings.[102] Approximately 57 percent of HSC transplant centers for adults offer outpatient transplants, although this is significantly less common among pediatric centers (19 percent).[103] For cord blood, approximately 97 percent of transplants occur in inpatient settings, according to our interviews. In Table 6.3, we present the percentage of transplants in each payer status (Medicare, Medicaid, and private payer) by transplant type and year for all inpatient discharges from the HCUP NIS data (see Chapter Three for more details). Although there is year-to-year variation and data suppression by HCUPnet, most of the inpatient transplants are covered by Medicaid or private insurers. We discuss typical coverage by private and public payers for transplants for both inpatient and outpatient transplants.

Medicaid

Medicaid is funded by both states and the federal government, but is administered by each state within federal guidelines. All states are required to cover low-income pregnant women, children through age 18, and typically also seniors or individuals with disabilities participating in the Supplemental Security Income program.

Similarly, state Medicaid programs are required to cover a certain set of services, but then states can cover additional services and have some latitude in determining the length and scope of services covered. Some states deliver Medicaid through a managed care program that receives a per-member-per-month payment for all services. Inpatient and outpatient hospital services are considered mandatory benefits, but states can decide whether and to what extent to cover HSC transplants as treatment and for which conditions.[104] A recent review of state Medicaid coverage found that all states report Medicaid coverage of HSC transplants, but the scope of coverage varied considerably.[104]

In Table 6.4, we present the average charges and costs for inpatient HSC transplants covered by Medicare and Medicaid based on HCUP data. Overall, Medicaid charges and costs tend to be higher than for Medicare. This may be driven by patient age if a large percentage of Medicaid patients is younger, because pediatric patients tend to require longer lengths of stay.

Medicare

Medicare covers individuals ages 65 and older who worked (and paid into the Medicare system for at least 10 years) and some younger individuals with disabilities or other conditions (e.g., end-stage renal disease, amyotrophic lateral sclerosis). Part A of Medicare covers inpatient care, including at hospitals, nursing homes, home health, and hospice. Part B covers care received in other settings (e.g., physician offices) and typically requires enrollees to pay a premium. Some Medicare beneficiaries choose to enroll in Medicare Advantage plans (also known as Part C), which combines Parts A and B into a plan administered by a private plan. Part D is optional and covers prescription drugs. Currently, Medicare covers allogeneic HSC transplants for

- leukemia, leukemia in remission, or aplastic anemia when it is reasonable and necessary
- severe combined immunodeficiency disease and Wiskott-Aldrich syndrome
- Myelodysplastic Syndromes pursuant to Coverage with Evidence Development (CED) in the context of a Medicare-approved, prospective clinical study.[105]

Table 6.3. Percentage of HSC Transplant Inpatient Stays Covered by Payers, 2005–2014

	41.03: Allogeneic Bone Marrow, No Purging (n = 9,200)			41.04: Autologous HSC, No Purging (n = 75,858)			41.05: Allogeneic HSC, No Purging (n = 39,822)			41.06: Cord Blood (n = 2,966)	
	Medicaid	Medicare	Private	Medicaid	Medicare	Private	Medicaid	Medicare	Private	Medicaid	Medicare
2005	21%	*	65%	62%	15%	*	67%	14%	*	*	38%
2006	57%	31%	*	58%	16%	*	70%	17%	*	*	*
2007	*	*	57%	8%	16%	65%	*		*	*	*
2008	73%	*	*	62%	12%	*	69%	13%	*	*	*
2009	63%	24%	*	12%	20%	64%	*	15%	*	*	*
2010	28%	*	59%	57%	14%	*	66%	15%	*	*	38%
2011	*	*	*	53%	12%	*	*	14%	*	*	*
2012	58%	23%	*	54%	10%	*	11%	17%	63%	63%	20%
2013	53%	26%	*	55%	12%	*	62%	12%	*	61%	*
2014	55%	25%	*	56%	11%	*	64%	10%	*	*	24%

SOURCE: HCUPnet 2005–2014 NIS (see Chapter Three).
NOTES: Cells with asterisks were suppressed by HCUPnet due to small sample sizes. No data were presented on private payers covering cord blood transplants. Note that the number of transplants does not match with our NMDP data because the HCUPnet NIS data are based on a 20-percent stratified sample of all discharges from U.S. community hospitals, excluding rehabilitation and long-term acute care hospitals.

Table 6.4. Average Hospital Charges and Costs Per Inpatient Stay in 2014, by Payer and Transplant Type

	Medicare		Medicaid	
	Charges	Costs	Charges	Costs
41.01: Autologous bone marrow transplant without purging	$184,390	$51,045	$230,799	*
	(18,218)	(4,378)	(61,984)	*
n	125		*	
41.03: Allogeneic bone marrow transplant without purging	$327,407	$114,503	$ 515,716	$180,426
	(59,850)	(25,326)	(68,302)	(25,007)
n	*		215	
41.04: Autologous HSC transplant without purging	$198,787	$53,322	$209,498	$60,119
	(13,574)	(3,015)	(14,481)	(4,064)
n	2,105		875	
41.05: Allogeneic HSC transplant without purging	$401,893	$112,012	$520,970	$164,143
	(28,422)	(7,011)	(45,876)	(16,246)
n	985		510	
41.06: Cord blood stem cell transplant	*$515,605*	*$149,864*	*$987,339*	*$296,896*
	(66,319)	*(20,224)*	*(252,707)*	*(71,633)*
n	*75*		*95*	

SOURCE: HCUPnet 2014 NIS (see Chapter Three).
NOTES: Standard errors in parentheses. Cells with asterisks were suppressed by HCUPnet due to small sample sizes. No cost or charge estimates for 41.06 in 2014 were available, so estimates (in italics) shown are 2013 values; all other values are from 2014. Sample sizes were too small to estimate costs and charges for ICD-9 code 41.08 (allogeneic HSC transplant with purging) by payer.

CMS has also proposed to expand coverage of HSC transplants pursuant to CED to multiple myeloma, myelofibrosis, and sickle cell disease.[106]

Inpatient Settings

Payment in inpatient settings tends to be based on diagnosis-related groups (DRGs) for both private and public payers. Medicare makes one diagnosis-specific payment for facility use that covers an entire hospital stay for up to 90 days (with some adjustments for type of hospital or other factors) as part of the Inpatient Prospective Payment System (IPPS).[a] Thus, in the case of HSC transplants, payment covers the cost of obtaining the donor cells as well as all labor, supplies, and drugs used during the treatment stay.

---

[a] Discharges are assigned to a DRG based on their principal diagnosis and up to 24 secondary diagnoses. DRG assignments can be influenced by patient age, gender, or discharge status. CMS uses the Medicare Severity DRG (MS-DRG) system, which is based on secondary diagnosis codes for major complication/comorbidity (MCC), complication/comorbidity (CC), or no complication/comorbidity (non-CC).[107]

Physicians typically bill for their services separately. For FY 2017, CMS reimburses $64,217 for allogeneic transplants (MS-DRG 014), $33,679 for autologous transplants when the patient has major comorbidities (MS-DRG 016), and $22,453 for autologous transplants when the patient does not have those comorbidities (MS-DRG 017) through IPPS.[108] The average hospital costs—according to the HCUP data for allogeneic transplants—ranges from $129,514 to $262,972 (for cord blood) (see Table 6.2). Analysis by the NMDP suggests that stem cell acquisition costs alone are $51,727 on average, or 81 percent of the total Medicare reimbursement.[97] However, acquisition costs vary considerably across states and by source. For example, cord blood and bone marrow acquisition costs in Colorado are estimated at $70,364 and $46,659, respectively, but are $45,863 and $67,246, respectively, in California.

Nonetheless, the total hospital cost estimates based on the HCUP data (Table 6.4) suggest that the current Medicare reimbursement does not fully cover the cost of HSC transplants. On average, the gap between reimbursement and hospital costs is largest for cord blood, but this may vary considerably by hospital.

Outpatient Settings

HSC transplants that occur in hospital outpatient departments are reimbursed by Medicare under the hospital Outpatient Prospective Payment System (OPPS). In OPPS, individual services are coded using the Healthcare Common Procedure Coding System, which are then assigned to ambulatory payment classifications (APCs). Payment is then calculated for each APC. Through 2016, HSC transplants were coded using APC 5281, apheresis and stem cell procedures, and the Medicare reimbursement rate was about $3,015 for all services. Acquisition costs for stem cells are the same regardless of whether the transplant occurs in an outpatient or inpatient setting. Thus, Medicare reimbursement for outpatient HSC transplants has historically covered less than 6 percent of the average stem cell acquisition costs of $51,727.

CMS proposed several new comprehensive APCs for 2017, including one for allogeneic HSC transplants (C-APC 5244), which will allow for future updating of the reimbursement rate based on provider cost reports that are specific to HSC transplants. The previously used code was also used by other unrelated and less costly services that pulled down the average costs and, thus, reimbursement. The proposed payment rate for C-APC is $15,267. Although this is significantly more than the previous reimbursement rate for outpatient HSC transplants, it is still considerably less than average acquisition costs. Some have argued that this lower reimbursement in outpatient settings may be incentivizing providers to choose more-expensive health care settings (e.g., inpatient) for HSC delivery.[97] One study comparing costs for 17 bone marrow transplant patients treated in outpatient settings with 115 patients treated in inpatient settings suggests lower charges for outpatient settings, but the extent to which Medicare beneficiaries were represented in this study is unclear.[93]

Private Payers

From discussions with key stakeholders and review of documents from a large insurance company, we found that allogeneic HSC transplantation is typically covered for certain conditions by private payers. Commercial or private payers tend to pay for inpatient HSC transplants based on a negotiated case rate that is typically bundled or episode-based, but the details of these contractual agreements between payers and transplant centers vary considerably. For example, the number of days after the transplant that are included in the bundle varies, and some transplant centers have negotiated a separate payment for cord blood on the basis that engraftment takes about ten days longer than for other HSC sources.

Some private payers will cover acquisition costs, though there may be limits. For example, for bone marrow donors, a patient may end up HLA-typing several potential family member donors to find a match, but acquisition costs may be capped at a certain dollar amount precluding coverage of typing multiple donors. Most private payers will not cover costs of private banking, often citing lack of support for this practice from the medical community.[74, 109–111]

Although a systematic accounting of private-payer coverage was not available, we found patient-level studies reporting a significantly greater likelihood of HSC transplantation among individuals covered by private insurance relative to public insurance (Medicaid or Medicare).[112, 113] However, it is unclear whether this is due to more-generous coverage benefits among the privately insured, better access to care, or other factors.

Evidence for Clinical Effectiveness

In this section, we highlight the status of the literature on the clinical effectiveness of different HSC sources; a full systematic review of this literature is beyond the scope of this study, but we aim to show how these factors tend to be considered for treatment decisions.

Overall, the evidence base for the clinical effectiveness of cord blood compared with bone marrow or peripheral blood is somewhat limited because there are currently no randomized trials comparing outcomes for HSC transplants using cord blood versus bone marrow or peripheral blood. There is one study currently under way with the potential to add significantly to the existing evidence—a multicenter randomized controlled trial comparing double cord blood transplants with haploidentical bone marrow transplants in patients with hematologic malignancies.[114] However, results from this study will not be available until 2019. In the meantime, we note that observational studies that have examined the clinical effectiveness of cord blood find that these treatments lead to comparable outcomes relative to alternative treatments.

We also note that older data comparing cord blood with bone marrow or peripheral blood often demonstrated worse post-transplant outcomes for CBUs. However, more-recent data tend to show similar outcomes for cord blood and bone marrow or peripheral blood. This change has been attributed to an increase in the minimum acceptable cell dose of the CBU to qualify for transplantation.[115]

One study compared outcomes of 450 patients receiving 5–6/6 HLA-matched unrelated donor transplants with 150 patients receiving 4–6/6 cord blood transplants.[116] Acute GVHD and relapse rates were similar between cord blood and 6/6 matched unrelated donor transplants, but patients who received matched unrelated donor transplants had better overall survival at three years (33 percent versus 23 percent) compared with patients who received 4–6/6 cord blood transplants. When cord blood was compared with 5/6 HLA-matched unrelated donor transplants, cord blood was shown to have a lower risk of acute GVHD but a similar risk of relapse, mortality, and disease-free survival.

A similar study compared outcomes of 682 adults with acute leukemia who received an HSC transplant: Ninety-eight patients received cord blood transplants and 584 patients were recipients of bone marrow transplants from an unrelated donor.[117] This study found that cord blood patients had a lower risk of GVHD and similar rates of relapse, mortality, and disease-free survival.

These findings were largely confirmed in a recent observational study that examined outcomes for 582 patients with either acute leukemia or myelodysplastic syndrome and minimal residual disease who received a primary HSC transplant from an unrelated cord blood donor (140 patients), an HLA-matched unrelated donor (344 patients), or an HLA-mismatched unrelated donor.[118] Compared with patients who received cord blood, patients who received an HLA-mismatched transplant had a greater risk of mortality within four years. For HLA-matched patients, there was no statistically significant difference in the risk of mortality within four years compared with cord blood patients. A closer examination of patients with minimal residual disease found that the risk of death in the HLA-mismatched group was even higher compared with the cord blood group. In patients without minimal residual disease at the time of transplant, HLA-mismatched patients still had a higher risk of mortality, but results were more comparable. Patients who received a cord blood transplant had lower rates of relapse than patients who received either an HLA-mismatched or an HLA-matched transplant. However, the results were only statistically significant for patients with a history of minimal residual disease prior to transplantation. Compared with patients who received a cord blood transplant, patients who received an HLA-mismatched transplant were 3.01 times more likely to relapse, while patients with an HLA-matched transplant were 2.92 times more likely to relapse. Overall, this study showed that cord blood performed similarly to HLA-matched unrelated donor sources and generally better than HLA-mismatched donor sources, particularly in the presence of minimal residual disease.

Another study examined children under the age of 16 with acute leukemia and compared 503 patients who received a cord blood transplant with 282 bone marrow transplant recipients.[119] For patients who received cord blood transplants with either one or two antigens mismatched, five-year survival rates were similar to those of HLA-matched bone marrow transplants. Mortality rates for matched cord blood transplants approached statistical significance for lower mortality rates than for matched bone marrow. Relapse rates were also similar when comparing allele-matched bone marrow with matched cord blood as well as cord blood with one antigen mismatch. For patients who received cord blood with two antigen mismatches, relapse rates were actually slightly lower compared with patients who received matched bone marrow.

In one study of 171 adults—some of whom received a single-CBU transplant (n = 100), some received 5–6/6 HLA-matched related donor bone marrow transplants (n = 55), and some received 5–6/6 HLA-matched related donor peripheral blood HSC transplants (n = 16)—patients who received cord blood demonstrated delayed hematologic recovery and a lower incidence of grade III–IV acute and extensive chronic GVHD compared with patients who received bone marrow or peripheral blood.[120] Cord blood and related donor transplantation had similar relapse, transplant-related mortality, and disease-free survival rates.

Overall, no recent studies have examined the clinical effectiveness of cord blood treatments compared with bone marrow or peripheral blood using randomized controlled trials. At least one important randomized controlled trial is under way,[114] however, and observational studies that have examined the clinical efficacy of cord blood compared with bone marrow or peripheral blood have generally found similar outcomes for most patients. Future studies may result in a shift in the balance of benefit versus risk for cord blood compared with bone marrow or peripheral blood. However, for the moment, the evidence currently supports the clinical effectiveness of cord blood compared with other HSC sources, particularly in the absence of a matched related donor source.

We note several general issues with comparing outcomes across these different HSC sources. First, selection of an HSC source is clearly nonrandom. Some of our key interviewees shared that CBUs are used only as a last resort, whereas others mentioned a preference for CBUs, particularly for certain types of patients. Patients at advanced stages of disease who do not have time to wait for a donor may be more likely to choose cord blood. Thus, any comparison of patients using different HSC sources suffers from this selection bias. Although this can be addressed, somewhat, by conducting randomized controlled trials, the sample would need to be restricted to patients for whom all sources are available, which limits the generalizability of findings. Second, the majority of the literature to date on clinical effectiveness follows patients for a relatively short time period. Because cord blood transplants take longer to engraft, examining outcomes over a short time frame will bias results toward more-favorable outcomes for other sources. Finally, even if CBUs yield better patient outcomes over the longer term, payer reimbursement preferences may render this moot. Specifically, because patients tend to change health insurance plans or coverage every few years, private insurers prefer to cover services that are less expensive in the short-to-medium term.

Summary

In this chapter, we examined the costs related to processing and banking CBUs and the revenue sources for CBBs. On average, the total variable costs per collected CBU range from $1,700 to $3,100. The average fee per unit used for transplant is $36,200. We also discussed other sources of revenue, including the HRSA subsidy, which, on average, is about $1,200 per unit listed on The Registry. In the next chapter, we use these costs and revenues—in conjunction with the NMDP data on units collected and shipped annually—to estimate CBB's break-even point.

Next, we discussed treatment costs from the payer's or patient's perspective. These costs include not only the cost of the HSC source (i.e., the cost of the CBU), but also the costs associated with the transplant, which most frequently occurs in an inpatient or hospital setting. The rules across payers vary, but we estimated that the average inpatient stay charge was $485,000, $571,000, and $831,000 for allogeneic transplants using bone marrow, peripheral blood stem cells, and cord blood, respectively. These treatments tend to occur over very different lengths of stay: 37.5, 33.5, and 51.2 days for bone marrow, peripheral blood stem cells, and cord blood, respectively.

Finally, we briefly reviewed the literature on the clinical effectiveness of HSC transplants. To date, there is not a single source that is the clear winner in terms of best outcomes for all patients. We discussed several issues with this literature, however, as selection of a stem cell source is clearly nonrandom and there has not been much evidence from longer-term outcomes that addresses the fact that cord blood transplant patients may simply take longer to heal initially due to the longer engraftment period.

Chapter Seven. Cord Blood Bank Financial Sustainability

In this chapter, we describe challenges and trade-offs that CBBs face while trying to optimize collection and banking of CBUs. We use standard economic theory of firm profit maximization to model how CBBs would behave in perfectly competitive markets. We use this analysis to provide a benchmark for consideration of how to potentially improve the financial sustainability of the banks in the industry with the caveat that the market for cord blood is likely not perfectly competitive. In economics, *profit maximization* means that the firm is breaking even or covering all its costs. As we discuss in Chapter Nine, the cord blood inventory can be thought of as a public good in that individuals derive value from its presence even when they are not explicitly using it (i.e., they know it is available to them if needed). Although many CBBs are part of larger corporate entities (i.e., hospitals, blood banks, or universities), we focus on one decision that each CBB makes: how many CBUs to collect and bank given HRSA's involvement in the market. We also briefly describe examples of alternative organizational structures to public cord blood banking and potential financial synergies between them.

CBBs' Collection Decisions

Public CBBs face the financial and logistical challenge of balancing the sometimes competing goals of maximizing CBU quality, diversity, and quantity. In the following sections, we describe and analyze the difficulties CBBs face in pursuing each of these goals.

TNC Count

TNC count is often used as measure of quality by CBBs because it is highly correlated with alternative measures of quality (such as CD34 or colony-forming unit counts), and therefore proxies for graft potency in the event of transplant.[121–126] Not surprisingly, the likelihood of both CBU use and transplant success is greatest among high–TNC count units.[81, 121, 127–129] Among all transplanted CBUs from NMDP data from 2007 to 2016, only 11 percent had a TNC count below 1.25×10^9 (see Figure 7.1). The share of transplanted CBUs, however, was 28 percent and 59 percent for CBUs with TNC counts of $1.25–1.75 \times 10^9$ and 1.75×10^9 or more, respectively. Thus, the release rate, calculated as the number of CBUs used divided by the total number of units banked, was also greater among higher–TNC count units (see the dotted line in Figure 7.1). This release rate is the highest (around 3 percent) for units with TNCs larger than 2.5×10^9. Because our bank-level data only report the number of units that are banked and shipped between 2010 and 2016, we are underestimating the actual inventory size for the number of units that were banked prior to 2010. Thus, release rates reported are likely an upper bound of actual release rates during this period.

Figure 7.1. Number of Banked CBUs and Release Rate, by TNC

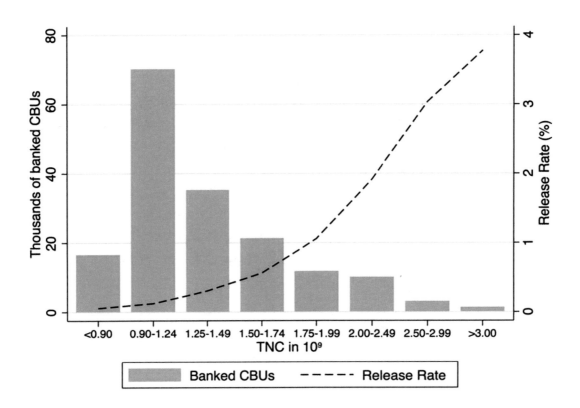

SOURCE: RAND authors' calculations using NDMP aggregated bank-level data for all 22 public banks in the United States between 2007 and 2016.
NOTES: The release rate is calculated as the ratio between the total number of shipped units and the number of banked units within each TNC group, divided by the ten years for which the data are available. Each bar represents the total number of CBUs banked by TNC group during 2007–2016. TNC is expressed in 10^9 units.

The incentive for storing high-quality CBUs is relatively high because the use of the higher–TNC count CBUs currently generates about 70 percent of public CBBs' revenue.[127] However, this could change if cord blood cell expansion technologies someday render smaller units more effective for transplantation (see Chapter Eight for further discussion of this future possibility).[127] Similar ratios of released units relative to the banked inventory are observed in other countries, such as France, Italy, Germany, and Australia.[130] These ratios are typically the smallest for banks with the largest inventories as a consequence of storing large numbers of low-quality units.

However, banking only units with higher TNCs is potentially problematic because TNC count is not observed until after a unit is collected. Therefore, focusing on banking

CBUs with higher TNC counts means that fewer collected units will ultimately be banked. In other words, the number of units discarded or not used for transplant will be higher if the bank focuses on high–TNC count units only. By *discarded*, we simply mean that the units were not banked; they may still have been used for research or other purposes. Based on an analysis of 1,839 CBUs collected by the Anthony Nolan Cell Therapy Centre (ANCTC), the population-average TNC count is estimated to be about 1.10×10^9, with a standard deviation of 0.65×10^9; the distribution is skewed toward lower TNC counts.[121] Thus, assuming a lognormal distribution implies that 40 percent of collected CBUs would not be banked if the TNC threshold matched the HRSA threshold of 9.0×10^9. A TNC threshold of 1.50×10^9 would yield a discard rate of 72 percent. These estimates are consistent with information we obtained from our interviews and from data provided by the NMDP. One interviewee suggested that a TNC threshold of 9.0×10^9 implied a discard rate of 67 percent. Another study suggested that if the TNC threshold was increased to 1.50×10^9, the discard rate would be 92 percent.[127] The difference between these discard rates may be driven by the fact that ANCTC has staff dedicated to CBU collection, potentially allowing for higher TNCs on average due to larger volumes.

Therefore, banks have to consider the trade-offs between having a higher release rate and higher–TNC count units and the number or rate of collected units that they will bank at the higher threshold. These concerns can be mitigated by ensuring that individuals collecting the CBUs are highly trained (training is correlated with collection of higher–TNC count units[131, 132]), or endeavoring to improve processing and reduction in waste of the already collected CBUs.[121]

The current structure of the NCBI program complicates this decision for banks because the program implicitly incentivizes the collection of lower–TNC count units by allowing CBBs to collect subsidies for banked units with TNC counts as low as 0.9×10^9. Indeed, among NCBI banks, the largest share—46.8 percent—of their banked NCBI units have a TNC count between 0.9 and 1.24×10^9 (see blue bars in Figure 7.2). These lower–TNC count units represent about one-third of all NCBI and non-NCBI units collected by the NCBI banks. However, for units with TNC counts above 1.25×10^9, the distribution of the CBU shares by TNC value is similar for both bank types and CBUs.

The minimum TNC value in some other countries is higher than what HRSA requires: 1.4×10^9 at the Anthony Nolan CBB in the United Kingdom and at Réseau Français du Sang Placentaire in France and 2.0×10^9 at the Barcelona CBB in Spain, for example.

Figure 7.2. Number of CBUs Banked by NCBI and Non-NCBI Banks, by TNC Count, 2007–2016

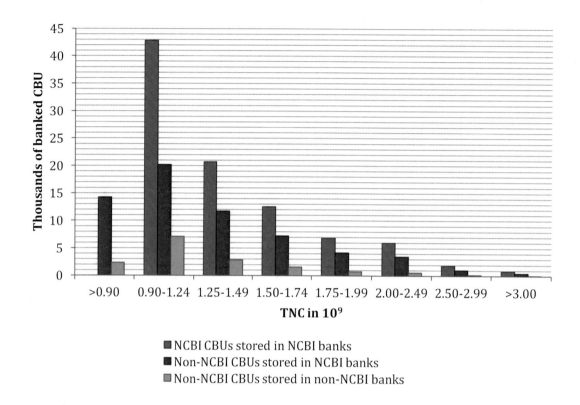

SOURCE: RAND authors' calculations based on NMDP bank-level data from 2007 to 2016.
NOTE: NCBI and non-NCBI banks can bank non-NCBI CBUs. TNC count is expressed in 10^9 units.

Inventory Size

Although a larger national inventory size can improve patient survival by increasing the likelihood that a transplant candidate will find a stored unit, the average costs incurred at the bank level for each additional CBU has been estimated at between $1,700 and $3,100 (see Table 6.1). On average, public CBBs collect about 8,500 CBUs annually, but ultimately bank far fewer CBUs. In our interviews with public CBB representatives, anywhere from 5 to 40 percent of the collected units are ultimately banked. Thus, for CBBs to break even, the HRSA subsidies received for all banked units and the fees collected from transplant centers for units used should ideally cover the costs of all the CBUs collected, including those that are discarded and in addition to the overhead costs per unit. Previous research using simulation models estimated that CBBs break even (assuming a national inventory level of 50,000 CBUs) when the fee charged to hospitals is approximately $15,000 per unit. To meet a larger national inventory of 150,000 units, it was then estimated that the break-even fee was around $46,000 per unit.[86] The difference is largely due to costs of collection that increase with inventory size.

72

Under the Stem Cell Therapeutic and Research Act, 150,000 units was the minimum number of new CBUs that NCBI aimed to add to the national inventory. As of 2016, the average public CBB's inventory was around 18,260, with nearly 200,000 CBUs across all public CBBs, although not all are part of NCBI. On average, the variable costs per shipped CBU at the industry level are similar to the fee per released unit that banks actually charge—between $29,000 and $45,000, which is consistent with earlier estimates.[86]

Diversity Challenge

Even with a current national inventory of over 200,000 CBUs, it remains challenging for minority patients to find a match. This is particularly true for some populations, such as African-Americans, Asians, and Southern Europeans—in part because of the relatively high number of rare HLA combinations that occurs in these groups.[16, 133] To ensure the increased representation of ethnic minorities on The Registry, priority funding from HRSA's NCBI program is directed toward collecting minority units, particularly from donors of Asian and African descent.[134]

NCBI subsidies provide between 10 and 35 percent of banks' total collection and processing costs according to our interview respondents and data provided by the NMDP. Thus, HRSA's NCBI funding is critical for banks and HRSA funding priorities strongly influence CBBs' collection strategies.[135] This has important financial implications for CBBs. First, as indicated in our qualitative data in Chapter Four, the collection of minority units is more challenging than collection of nonminority units. Cord blood programs routinely recruit pregnant women in doctors' offices and in prenatal classes, which minorities are statistically less likely to receive. Many minority groups also learn too late in the prenatal process about the possibility of donation. Some believe that cord blood donation is costly (although public donation is free) or they mistakenly believe it will hurt the newborn.[136, 137] For these and other reasons, fewer minority mothers have been banking cord units.[138]

Some studies suggest that CBUs from minority donors may be smaller by some measures (TNC count, volume, CD34+ count) compared with CBUs from Caucasian donors, but others suggest no correlation between TNC count and volume in preprocessed or postprocessed units and race or ethnicity.[132, 138, 139] Although data on collected CBUs were not available to us, we showed in Chapter Five that there is some variation in TNC count across race or ethnicity in both banked and shipped CBUs.

Based on NMDP data, about 42 percent of African-American patients are matched with donors of African descent. Yet the probability that they are matched with Caucasian donors increases with increasing TNC count (see Figure 7.3). For instance, among African-American patients treated with CBUs with TNC counts between 0.9 and 1.24×10^9, only 16 percent of donor units were from Caucasian patients. However, among those treated with higher–TNC count units, between 30 and 37 percent were matched to a Caucasian donor.

However, increasing the TNC count cannot overcome large HLA mismatches. Only between 1 and 17 percent of the U.S. population can find a CBU with no HLA mismatches, whereas 81–96 percent can find a unit with one or two HLA mismatches, depending on their race/ethnicity.[140] One study found that in cases where there were one or 2 two HLA mismatches, the best patient outcomes (lowest mortality rates) were from units with TNC counts higher than 5.0×10^7 per kg as compared to dosing of 2.5×10^7 or less.[141] An average-weight adult male would need a CBU with a TNC count of at least 4.40×10^9, whereas an average-weight adult female would need a CBU with a TNC count of at least 3.75×10^9. The implication is that, unless cell expansion technologies solve this problem, banks should focus on collecting CBUs with higher TNC counts as one strategy to improve genetic diversity because they can offset the detrimental effects of HLA mismatches. There is still a significant percentage of minority groups for whom acceptable units are not available.

Figure 7.3. Donor's Race/Ethnicity for African-American Cord Blood Transplant Patients, by TNC Count

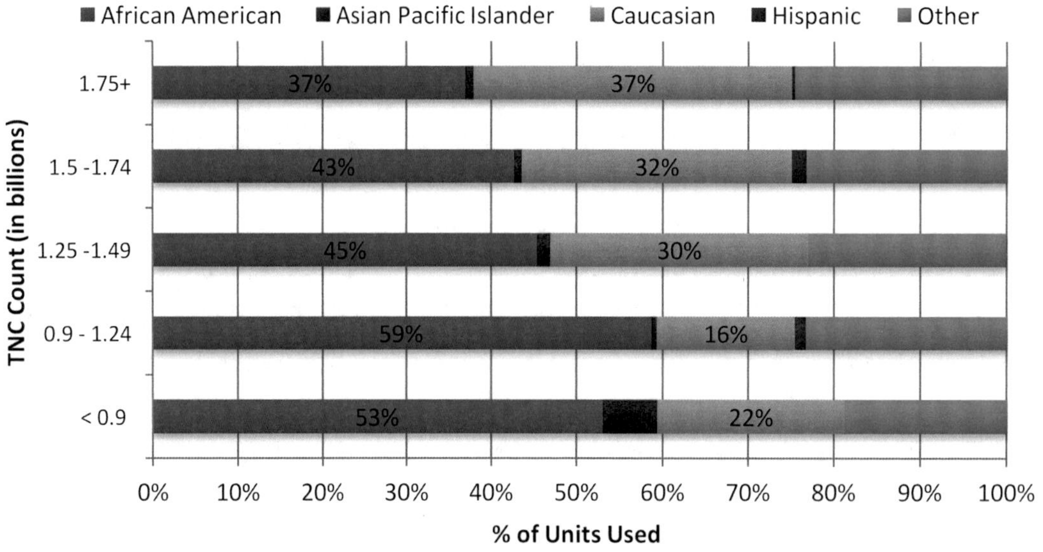

SOURCE: RAND authors' calculations based on NMDP data for matches between donors and patients between 2010 and 2016.
NOTE: Patterns are similar for other races/ethnicities (see Table C.1 in Appendix C for additional results).

Despite the ability to overcome mismatches by increasing TNC counts, banking additional minority units is still critical. Some researchers have suggested that public CBBs should not restrict the CBUs for banking by initial TNC levels, but rather rely on analyzing the HLA type before discarding units with low TNC counts to ensure their inventory's racial/ethnic diversity.[142]

To optimize their business processes and to qualify for the HRSA NCBI subsidies, public CBBs that we interviewed often set different thresholds for banking minority (as high as 1.25×10^9) and Caucasian CBUs (as high as 1.80×10^9). Some banks only pursue NCBI subsidies for non-Caucasian units.

A representative from one bank suggested that banking minority units should be centralized in large minority hospitals, with more than 10,000 minority births per year, rather than spread through many smaller banks. One study shows that racial diversity can be achieved in a national network of CBBs by focusing collections in specific geographic areas.[138] Detroit, for example, has the highest percentage of African-American donors and San Diego has the highest percentage of Hispanic donors, so some have suggested that collections should be focused accordingly.[142]

CBBs' Financial Decisions: How to Break Even

In this section, we considered two approaches to estimate the break-even price and quantity for public CBBs. Although public CBBs are typically nonprofits and the CBUs are donated freely by altruistic donors, they still need to be able to cover their costs to stay in operation. Thus, our calculations here are intended to determine the extent to which CBBs are able to cover their costs given current costs and banking statistics. First, we used average total variable costs as delineated in Chapter Six, along with the actual quantities of CBUs shipped (transplanted), by TNC count. From our interviews and NMDP data, we then constructed an average variable cost per shipped unit to compare to the average fee CBBs receive from hospitals. Second, we used a more formal profit maximization model (presented in Appendix B), where we accounted for the differing discard rates, as well as the varying probability that a given collected CBU would have a particular TNC count. We then used the average variable cost measures as reported in Table 6.1 in Chapter Six to estimate the bank-level equilibrium quantity of units to collect.

Estimating the Break-Even Price: Comparing Variable Cost and Fee per Shipped CBU

In Chapter Six, we reported details on average variable costs for CBBs across various stages of the process of collecting, testing, processing, and storing CBUs. The average total variable cost for a collected unit ranged between $1,700 and $3,100, with about $1,300 going toward costs accrued prior to releasing the unit for transplant (see Table 6.1). For this reason, we estimated break-even numbers using variable costs per unit of $1,300 and $3,100 to obtain a reasonable range of estimates. As we detail below, less than 3 percent of collected units are ultimately used for transplant, although this varies considerably by the TNC count of the unit.

We calculated the average variable cost *per unit shipped,* allowing it to vary by TNC count due to the differences in the probability of use. As expected, the average variable cost per unit shipped declines with TNC count because more of the higher–TNC count units are shipped. For example, the average variable cost per unit shipped ranges from about \$3,100 to \$7,300 for NCBI units with a TNC count higher than 3.0×10^9 relative to about \$102,000 to \$240,000 for NCBI units with a TNC count between 0.9 and 1.24×10^9. Non-NCBI units cost slightly more per unit. This is driven by the release rates, not by collection costs. The cost per shipped unit across all TNC counts is \$29,000 and \$67,000, assuming a variable cost of \$1,300 and \$3,100 per unit collected, respectively. This range is consistent with what has been reported elsewhere and with the fees CBBs charge transplant centers (the average fee is \$36,200).[127]

Comparing the variable cost per unit shipped to the expected revenue per unit shipped provides an estimate of the bank's break-even point—that is, the price and quantity of units sold that would allow the bank to cover all its variable costs. For this analysis, we assumed that banks do not charge hospitals differentially based on TNC count. Using the average transplant fee per shipped CBU of \$36,200, we found that banks only break even at TNC levels higher than 1.50×10^9 and 1.75×10^9 on NCBI and non-NCBI units, respectively (see Figure 7.4). Using the actual number of units shipped by TNC count and average variable costs, our analysis suggests that banks mostly lose money on lower–TNC count units. On average, we estimated that the overhead cost per banked CBU is around \$1,560. Factoring this cost into the analysis yields a total cost per shipped CBU of \$62,000 to \$101,000, depending on the assumed variable cost (\$1,300 or \$3,100). For CBBs with TNC-count thresholds below 1.50×10^9, the difference between revenues from transplant fees for units shipped and the total variable and overhead costs for all collected units is negative.

Estimating the Break-Even Price: Economic Model of Profit Maximization

In this section, we used a standard economic model that assumes that the bank will seek to collect as many units at a given sales price to maximize their profits (see Appendix B for more details). However, we assumed the TNC count of any given unit follows the probability that a randomly chosen unit has that TNC count. For example, based on the literature, the probability that a randomly drawn unit will have a TNC count of less than 0.9×10^9 is 0.40 (40 percent), whereas the probability that a given unit will have a TNC count of more than 1.75×10^9 is 0.21 (21 percent) (see Table 7.1). Then, based on actual banking and shipment quantities from the NMDP, we assumed that the probability that a collected unit is banked and shipped varies depending upon the TNC count, as shown in Table 7.1. For example, the probability that a CBU with a TNC count

76

between 0.9 and 1.24×10^9 will be *banked* if the bank's threshold is 0.9 is 0.35, but the probability that it would actually be *used* is only 0.0012 (0.12 percent).The probability that a CBU with a TNC count of more than 1.75×10^9 will be *banked* under the current minimum threshold reimbursable by HRSA is between 0.05 and 0.12 (a 5- to 12-percent chance in a given year), whereas the probability that it will be *used* is between 1 and 4 percent per year.

Using these assumptions and the average variable costs as delineated in Chapter Six, we estimated the total costs and revenues for banks allowing for differing internal TNC-count thresholds. Consistent with other studies, we found that, on average, public CBBs that bank only units with higher TNC counts generate greater profits, even after taking into account the lower probability of being able to collect those units (see Table 7.2).

Figure 7.4. Break Even: Total Variable Cost per Shipped Units Relative to Fee per Shipped Units

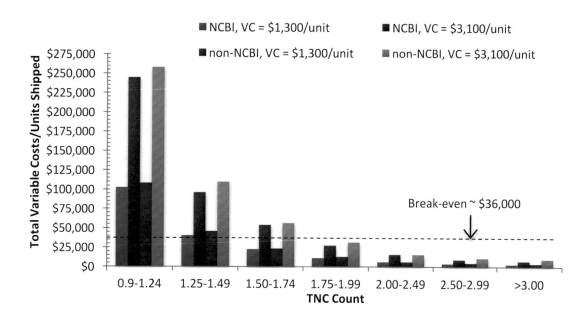

SOURCE: RAND authors' calculations based on the assumption of $1,300 or $3,100 in variable costs per unit and actual number of units shipped (both NCBI and non-NCBI) from NMDP data between 2007 and 2016.
NOTE: TNC count is expressed in 10^9 units. VC = variable cost.

Summary

In this chapter, we described key challenges that public CBBs face while trying to optimize collection and banking of CBUs. The first challenge is the CBB's decision on what *quality-level* (TNC count) CBUs to bank. On the one hand, we found that the likelihood that CBUs will be used for transplant increases with TNC count. Among all CBUs used for transplants from 2007 to 2016, only 11 percent had a TNC count below

1.25×10^9 and, in a given year, the probability that such a unit would be used is approximately one-tenth of 1 percent. Among all CBUs used for transplant over the same period, about 61 percent had a TNC count higher than 1.5×10^9. The release rate—or the ratio of units shipped to units available in inventory—is highest for units with a TNC count higher than 2.5×10^9, at around 3 percent. On the other hand, collecting high-quality units is costly. In addition to lower costs, the current structure of the NCBI program implicitly incentivizes the collection of lower–TNC count units by allowing CBBs to collect subsidies for banked units with TNC counts as low as 0.9×10^9.

Second, CBBs must decide *how many* CBUs they will bank. Although a larger national inventory increases the likelihood that a transplant candidate can find a match with a stored unit, the average costs incurred at the bank level for each additional CBU is high. We estimated that, currently, the average public CBB's inventory is around 18,260, with nearly 200,000 CBUs in the national inventory in total, which is greater than the 150,000 that has been estimated as the optimal size, based on diversity and cost considerations.

The third challenge refers to CBBs' decisions to target racial/ethnic minority cord blood donors. To ensure increased representation of ethnic minorities listed on The Registry, priority funding from HRSA's NCBI program is directed toward collecting minority CBUs, particularly from Asians and African-Americans. Collecting minority units is challenging both because minorities are less likely to donate and because there is some evidence that minority units are smaller for biological reasons. We observed, however, that the probability that minority patients are matched with donors of the same race decreases with TNC count. This, in conjunction with evidence from other studies, suggests that that CBU size may be used to compensate for some level of HLA mismatching.

In the second part of this chapter, we estimated the profit maximization strategy for public CBBs. We estimated that the cost per shipped CBU is between $29,000 and $67,000. However, these costs vary significantly with TNC count; costs per shipped unit are below $10,000 for units with a TNC count higher than 3.0×10^9, and above $100,000 for those with a TNC count below 1.24×10^9. Finally, we estimated the total costs and revenues for banks allowing for differing internal TNC-count thresholds. We found that, on average, banks that bank only units with higher TNC counts generate greater profits, even after taking into account the lower probability of being able to collect those units.

Table 7.1. Probability CBU Will Be Collected, Banked, and Shipped, by TNC Count

TNC Count	Collected	Banked if TNC threshold is:							Shipped
		0.90	1.25	1.50	1.75	2.00	2.50	3.00	
Less than 0.90	0.40	0.00	0.00	0.00	0.00	0.00	0.00	0	0.0056
0.9–1.24	0.21	0.35	0.00	0.00	0.00	0.00	0.00	0	0.0012
1.25–1.49	0.12	0.20	0.31	0.00	0.00	0.00	0.00	0	0.0031
1.50–1.74	0.06	0.10	0.15	0.22	0.00	0.00	0.00	0	0.0056
1.75–1.99	0.06	0.10	0.15	0.22	0.29	0.00	0.00	0	0.0106
2.00–2.49	0.07	0.12	0.18	0.26	0.33	0.47	0.00	0	0.0192
2.50–2.99	0.03	0.05	0.08	0.11	0.14	0.20	0.38	0	0.0304
More than 3.00	0.05	0.08	0.13	0.19	0.24	0.33	0.63	1	0.0378

SOURCE: RAND authors' calculations.
NOTES: The *Collected* column reflects the probability that a given unit collected will have the corresponding TNC count (thus, column equals 1). The *Banked if TNC threshold is:* columns reflects the probability that a unit with a given TNC count will be banked, which is conditional on the unit being collected. This probability depends on what the bank's TNC threshold is (which we vary from 0.90 to 3.0 billion). Finally, the *Shipped* column reflects the probability that a unit with a given TNC count will be shipped for transplant. TNC counts are expressed in 10^9 units.

Table 7.2. Revenue, Cost, and Profit for CBBs, by Bank's Internal TNC Threshold

	Internal TNC Threshold						
	0.90	1.25	1.50	1.75	2.00	2.50	3.00
Total revenue	$6,204,833	$9,112,802	$12,280,778.58	$14,748,033	$17,904,774	$22,696,911	$24,499,335
Total cost	$10,753,722	$8,698,662	$7,524,342	$6,937,182	$6,350,022	$5,665,002	$5,371,422
Profit	−$4,548,888	$414,140	$4,756,436	$7,810,851	$11,554,752	$17,031,909	$19,127,913

SOURCE: RAND authors' calculations.
NOTE: TNC counts are expressed in 10^9 units.

Chapter Eight. Factors Shaping the Public Cord Blood Sector's Future

In Chapter Four, we identified and explained trends that have already affected the public cord blood system, and in this chapter we identify and analyze nascent or potential developments that could have a significant future impact on the sector. Because this chapter focuses on the future, it is by nature less certain and more speculative. We discuss and analyze possible developments that could either support or harm the cord blood sector.

Key Inputs to the Cord Blood Sector Are Reliable

We reviewed factors that are likely to support the growth or the financial stability of the cord blood system. Cord blood–sector stakeholders expressed confidence that future disruptions in the supply or availability of key inputs are highly unlikely. Such key inputs include umbilical cord and placenta donations and essential goods, equipment, and services. The available supply of new cord donations is likely to remain plentiful because the number of cord donations far outpaces the number required to sustain the sector. Furthermore, once cord blood is donated, processed, and stored, CBUs have a long shelf life relative to whole blood or other organs, for example. This makes the sector resistant to supply-side shocks when compared with other health sectors, such as whole blood, which requires a continuous resupply of perishable donations. For example, if an event were to temporarily disrupt a region's donation hospitals or shipping networks, this would not have a significant impact on the overall pipeline of CBUs available for transplantation.

The equipment and services required to maintain the cord blood sector are also reliable, in part because most of the sector's equipment and service providers do not rely exclusively or even primarily on sales to this sector. Several key suppliers to CBBs confirmed that they do not rely on public cord blood to sustain their businesses. For example, one leader of a blood-testing lab explained

> …cord blood testing is a tiny part [of our business]…less than 2 percent of our total samples tested per year. All [infectious disease] tests we do for CBBs are the same tests we do for our other clients. If the cord blood market collapsed it wouldn't affect us—we'd be testing the same markers in either method [cord blood or haploidentical].

Most components in cord collection kits are standard off-the-shelf medical supplies, with the exception of a cord blood collection bag. Cord blood processing equipment is specialized, but CBBs can choose from several suppliers. When asked whether there is any danger of exiting the market for cord blood processing equipment, one chief executive officer (CEO) explained

"...there is no danger of that. We are actually launching new technology to help the industry to grow."

He also explained that, despite the fact that cord blood processing machines represent a small portion of his company's overall sales, these machines use the same technology platform as other machines for point-of-care application and for immune oncology. This is yet another example of how the cord blood sector benefits from supplies, services, and infrastructure built for other medical sectors. Furthermore, even if machines to automate cord blood processing were to somehow become unavailable, CBBs can also function quite well without such equipment, and some choose to keep their processes manual because they believe they can achieve higher-quality CBUs using manual processes.

Considering all the above factors, public CBBs appear to enjoy a stable and predictable market for their key inputs. We assess the probability of a disruption in key inputs to be extremely low.

Other Types of Cord Blood Banks

Private Banks

The private cord banking sector interacts with and supports public banking and the broader market in several ways. Although public CBBs supply the overwhelming majority of CBUs that are actually transplanted, private CBBs still play a significant role in the system because they collect, process, and bank more than half of all CBUs in the world.[143] Furthermore, despite having a lower rate of transplantation, the private family banking market depends on and contributes to most of the same infrastructure that public CBBs require. For example, a representative of a private CBB shared about supporting education and outreach programs that also benefit public CBBs.

> We are supportive of public banks. For example, we have a public banking partner...an educational partnership.... As part of that partnership, we developed a [public] educational resource.... We have also provided grant funding to Be The Match® in support of the development of a webinar for [health care] professionals on CBB—public and private.

Private banks also invest considerable resources in advertising and marketing the benefits of banking cord blood and tissues to patients, and this investment likely produces positive spillover effects benefitting public CBBs by raising general awareness and understanding. Public CBBs generally lack funding for marketing, and mainly rely on hospital staff, websites, and brochures to inform and recruit potential donors. In contrast, private CBBs spend a significant amount of money on marketing.[32] Expectant mothers often see advertisements and brochures about cord blood that are typically produced by the private banks in their obstetricians' offices.

There is also evidence that private banks sometimes create new manufacturing techniques and processes that can benefit the public cord blood sector. A representative of a private CBB explained

> [w]e've had representatives from a variety of public banks, say the majority in the U.S., visit our lab over the last ten years. We've taken them on tours, discussed processes, best practices, and had good knowledge sharing.... Within the U.S., the family [private] banks were the first to initiate the cord tissue storage.

A manager in a hybrid CBB shared examples of innovations that started in private banks and could spread to public CBBs. This hybrid CBB is the only CBB in the United States that processes and stores placenta blood and tissue, an innovation that was funded by the private side of the hybrid bank. She also explained that

> [p]rivate banks...are providing the materials for what we call autologous transplants and cell therapies—for a child using their own stem cells. That could go on to become an allogeneic process—and the public banks could benefit from that as well.... There is a great interaction between public and private in that way. The privates are really supporting the cell therapy clinical trials using the autologous cord blood.

Some public banks derive significant income from private CBBs that contract with them to process and store private CBUs.[144] Representatives from several public banks that we interviewed confirmed that such contractual relationships are an important source of revenue and contribute to their financial sustainability.

Occasionally, the financial support that private CBBs provide to the cord blood market is indirect. For example, a supplier to both public and private CBBs stated that the business he generates from selling to private CBBs allows him to sell to public CBBs. This essentially means that the private side may be indirectly cross-subsidizing the public side. He explained

> [w]e don't make a lot [of money] from the donor industry [public CBBs]...what pays our rent are the private banks.

Although private banks help public CBBs in numerous ways, their influence is not always positive. As we described in Chapter Two, interviewees raised several concerns about the practices some private banks employ, and, more generally, there was concern from public banks and some practitioners about the role of private banks in the industry.

Hybrid and Alternative Cord Blood Banking Models

As discussed in earlier chapters, a few public U.S. CBBs have embraced a hybrid model, combining a public and private CBB within a single business entity. Such hybrid models allow public CBBs to spread the fixed costs of maintaining equipment, personnel, and facilities for collection, processing, and storage between their private and public operations.[134, 145] Since both public and private CBBs exist under a single organization, this allows the private banking to essentially subsidize the public banking component.

Several CBB representatives said that hybrid banks are attractive because the private side can compensate for the financial losses incurred on the public side. One manager in a hybrid CBB stated that

> [i]t's fair to say we'd never make a profit on the public side—it is a loss every year—we absorb that and we recognize that for what it is.... This was never profit-driven and [we] never sought to make money off of this [public banking]. The draw to this was to give back, because I don't think anyone believes you can make money with public banking.

Another manager of a different hybrid bank said

> [w]e started as a hybrid bank to get financial support for the public bank.... Public banking isn't profitable. Because of the private banking, I'm able to generate revenue to cover [public banking] expenses or losses.

Among public CBBs that are not hybrids, some are considering the option. One manager of a public CBB stated that

> [w]e have reached out to the community to look into setting up a private banking program to subsidize the public banking program.

In addition to hybrid models that are already helping public banking in the United States, there are other public-private partnership models that exist abroad, some of which U.S. banks may someday attempt to emulate. In such models, privately stored CBUs are made available to the public in one of three ways. First, it may be required by law that a certain share of otherwise privately stored units is donated for public use. A second approach is the so-called *hybrid split* or *dual banking*, in which the CBB splits a single CBU into two parts: One usually larger share of the CBU can be used for family and the other is stored for public use. The third approach is the so-called *hybrid requisition*, whereby parents pay for a CBU's storage but are either obliged or have an option to donate their privately stored cord blood in the event that someone else needs their unit. If a graft is used, the parents are reimbursed.[134, 146] These banks increase the inventory size of CBUs for public use, and thereby their utilization rates and revenues, improving public banks' finances.[146] This type of model does not exist in the United States because regulations for private and public CBBs are different. Thus, a unit that is collected and stored in a private CBB cannot move into public CBB registries.

There are several examples of these alternative models. Some examples from abroad are Eticur in Germany, Eurocord in Slovakia, Cryosave in Belgium, and Precious Cells Biobank in the United Kingdom.[148] The latter, for instance, offers fee-based cord blood storage, but also operates the Precious Cells Miracle, a charity that accepts free cord blood donations. Another example of this hybrid model is the China Cord Blood Corporation, of which the public banking division receives no government funding, despite being the largest public CBB in China.[149] In China, all CBBs are required by law to be hybrid. In the United States, UMass Memorial Medical Center in Worcester, Massachusetts, is a good example of a public CBB that transformed into a hybrid model to avoid closure.[145] This public CBB filed for bankruptcy in

2003 because the release rate, at less than 2 percent, was too small to cover its annual operating costs.[145] It was acquired by Lifeforce Cryobanks in 2006 and now offers storage at several collection sites across the United States.[146]

In Turkey, a certain share of otherwise privately stored units is required to be donated for public use, which results in 25 percent of all privately stored units being donated for public use. The Virgin Health Bank established in 2007 in the United Kingdom is an example of a hybrid split bank that pioneered the 20-to-80 hybrid model, where 20 percent of the CBU volume was stored for private use and 80 percent was stored for public use.[27, 150] Although the 20-percent CBU share is insufficient for a successful transplant, the hope was that cell expansion could be used to regenerate its volume to a useable amount. This technology is still in experimental stages. However, in 2009, the Virgin Health Bank had to change its business model to avoid bankruptcy. Finally, examples of the requisition approach can be found in Spain and Germany, where parents are obliged to donate their privately stored cord blood or have an option to donate it, respectively.[134, 146]

Potential Changes Affecting the Selection of HSC Sources

As explained in Chapters One and Four, the U.S. cord blood sector currently functions inside a larger market for HSCs that also includes bone marrow and peripheral blood. In recent years, the share of HPC transplants that used haploidentical sources has been rising (see Text Box 3 in Chapter Four), while the share of CBU transplants has fallen, both in the United States and abroad.[151] In this section, we explore the potential for further growth in the relative number of haploidentical HSC transplants, which might contribute to lower demand for cord blood and increasing financial pressure on CBBs.

Investments in infrastructure and training that support haploidentical transplants and reduced investments in cord blood infrastructure and training may be self-perpetuating. This market momentum may weigh significantly in the calculations that transplantation specialists make when selecting one HSC source over another.

For example, an increasing number of transfusion specialists may choose haploidentical sources of HSCs mainly because they have more experience with haploidentical sources or no experience with cord blood. As one transfusion specialist explained,

> [y]ou will speak to transplant physicians who won't do cords; end of discussion. If you don't have experience with cords or limited and unsuccessful experience, their reluctance stands to reason.

As one leader of a hybrid CBB elaborated,

> [t]he problem will be when the market collapses and there are new people coming in that are training in haploidentical, etc., not cord blood—it will take 20 years to reboot the [cord blood] training—you can't get the trained people back if you are not doing these types of transplants—even though with cord blood you have the best outcomes.

Falling cord blood sales could also motivate CBBs to recover costs by raising prices, and higher prices could perpetuate further reductions in the quantity of CBUs demanded. Increased volume of collection, processing, and increased purchases of equipment used for haploidentical collections, processing, and transfusions could lower the price of haploidentical options and perpetuate the fall in demand for cord blood.

In contrast, new innovations and technologies that boost the relative efficacy of cord blood or other HSC sources may impact demand for cord blood in the opposite direction. For example, some promising new technologies and techniques aim to increase CBU cell counts by expanding cells within a CBU or by combining multiple CBUs. Other researchers are exploring reduced-intensity (nonmyeloablative) stem cell transplantation preparative regimens, or combining expanded or otherwise altered HSCs with normal CBUs to improve grafting speed, donor-recipient compatibility, and immune system development.[152] If proven successful, any of these new techniques could improve the demand for cord blood by increasing its efficacy, particularly with larger (adult) patients.

Potential Changes Affecting the Use of Cord Blood

In-vitro cell expansion techniques that increase the TNC count of a CBU have recently been tested by biotechnology companies, including Nohla Therapeutics, NiCord, Gamida, and others. Nohla pioneered using expanded CBUs to improve patient survival before HSCs finish engrafting and taking on blood system functions.[153] These expanded cells can be transplanted alongside an HLA-matched CBU to help support the patient's immune system while the HLA-matched CBU engrafts.

One stem cell scientist expressed some optimism that HSC expansion technology could begin to increase demand for CBUs during the next three to five years. He explained that

> [t]he last two years have seen some significant work at [the University of Minnesota], a group in Canada, and Peter Rossi's work in Boston set up by Third Rock Ventures. All three have shown significant expansion without the loss of engraftment ability. It still needs to be validated. Could be a real game-changer in the industry.

A manager of a hybrid bank and a partner corporation explained another new technology that can be used both for growing MSCs for diabetic wound healing or for growing HSCs. The CBB manager explained that

> ...we don't know if we can grow long-term grafting cells, but we probably can. A lot of cells can be grown in these hollow fibers—that [is] a great technology with easy expansion capability that open[s] things tremendously, whereas growing in a flask isn't easy.

Although expansion technology could increase the demand for the many banked CBUs that are currently too small for transplantation, there remains the danger that these technologies may not develop quickly enough to help existing CBBs. One HSC transplantation specialist opined that

> …at least two-thirds of the [already-banked cord blood] units are useless [currently too small for transplantation] and expansion technology isn't there yet. The [cord blood transplantation] field will be gone before expansion is big enough.

Although expansion technologies could help the cord blood sector, other changes in technology could someday severely disrupt or replace the existing cord blood system. After several decades of research,[154] during the past five years a few biotechnology companies have made significant progress in propagating or expanding HSCs,[155] as discussed earlier in this chapter. On the one hand, moderate success in this field greatly benefits the cord blood sector in that it can help small CBUs to effectively treat adult patients. However, if farther into the future this same technology reaches the point where lines of HSCs can be indefinitely cultured in-vitro, as is currently done with some embryonic stem cell lines, total demand for units banked in CBBs could dramatically fall.

Potential New Clinical Applications for Cord Blood

Several potential new clinical applications for cord blood are under development. Success in these trials could open up new potential applications for CBUs. A prominent researcher who uses cord blood noted that

> [t]he stem cell industry…is an amazing industry to be in. There are companies all the time being formed. Some of the regenerative medicine is coming out of cord blood. There is concern that once these industries take off, we'll hit [use up] the [cord blood] inventory very hard.

A manager of a hybrid CBB added that

> [t]he [cord blood] market is pretty plateaued—but, with the promise of regenerative medicine and cell therapy and what we are seeing today—we could, if we had one breakthrough in cell therapy using cord blood—which is a couple of phase II clinical trials—if we have one breakthrough with these common diseases—for instance—stroke, cerebral palsy, autism, then I think we will see exponential growth. I think it is really going to depend on clinical trials.

> The private [CBBs] are really supporting the cell therapy clinical trials using the autologous cord blood…for cerebral palsy for instance there have been two clinical trials—one using a child's own autologous cord blood, and one using a sibling's cord blood. [This] might go on to be another reason for public banks to release units.

A CEO of a private bank concurred that

> [t]here are some promising studies from Duke on [cerebral palsy, traumatic brain injury], and autism—we are hearing good results—and these studies need to be published—and hopefully moved to the FDA.

A biotechnology venture from Cellectis is looking at CAR T-cell therapy. According to a prominent stem cell scientist,

> [t]he best source of off-the-shelf T-cells, which you don't have to match, would be cord blood. That would increase the demand for small CBUs.

We do note that organizations that depend on cord blood sales may be exhibiting bias when expressing optimism about the prospects of new medical applications for cord blood. Because we primarily interviewed people whose careers depend on the growth of cord blood sector for this study, we must interpret these findings with caution.

Cord Blood Banks Could Bank Other Stem Cells and Tissues

Beyond cord blood, other cells and tissues derived from cords and placentas could also yield new medical applications, and CBBs may be well positioned to participate in any new markets that arise. Neonatal tissues are also a source of MSCs, discussed in Chapter Two, and other cells that have many potential therapeutic applications. Because CBBs have already established the infrastructure, expertise, and relationships to collect neonatal tissue donations, CBBs would be well suited to take advantage of any new demand for related tissues. One CEO of a company that supplies equipment to various medical sectors explained

> [y]ou're seeing a predominant number of trials in recent years that are focused on mesenchymal stem cells. It's a global trend. And if you're looking at how many stem cell…technologies have been approved globally, it's about ten. And if you count what are really the cells that are being used or approved, you will see that nine out of ten were approved for MSC and only one for cord blood. So that gives you a sense of where the industry is and is going.

New demand for neonatal cells and tissues could allow CBBs to expand their businesses and achieve greater efficiencies of scale in the collection, transportation, testing, processing, and storage of neonatal tissues and cells. Whereas CBBs currently discard the vast majority of donations because they do not meet the requirements specific to cord blood and HSC transplantation, additional uses for cord tissues and placentas would allow at least some currently discarded donations to go toward productive uses. Additionally, there could be some donations that yield both cord blood and other useful cells, and, in such cases, the costs of collection, transportation, and disease testing would be shared between the cord blood and other products, thereby lowering cord blood costs per unit and improving CBB profit margins.

Many private CBBs already collect and store MSCs and tissues in addition to cord blood, and these private CBBs could quickly transfer this knowledge to public CBBs via existing hybrid bank ownership structures and ongoing knowledge-sharing platforms. At least one hybrid CBB is already collecting and processing cord tissue for its private banking clients, and one hybrid CBB already has experience collecting placentas and harvesting their stem cells for private banking clients. A manager from a public CBB stated that her organization

...did invest for a number of years in experimenting with other populations of cells...particularly MSC and [natural killer] cells, but without funds to continue that research we had to stop.

Such experience could give some CBBs a head start in any potential new market for additional neonatal cells and tissues. As a representative of a private CBB explained,

> [y]ou see this anecdotally at medical conferences and in sidebar conversations...you hear that public banks have an interest in getting into cord tissue. I think it's only a matter of time before they start to take a look at that. There is a lot of exciting research with the mesenchymal stem cells. As the use of cord blood declines for transplant applications, and these public banks have a sizable amount of inventory collected for that use, they are looking for other avenues in the bio economy that they can use for a revenue source. I think you see Natera coming into the marketplace and their partnership with BloodWorks Northwest and Natera using the BloodWorks lab—you can imagine in collecting the cord tissue that there could be some things learned for BloodWorks that they could apply down [the] line.

Although some CBBs may be well positioned to expand into new markets, the FDA and other federal regulators may impede their rapid expansion into the collection and storage of new cell types. Many federal regulations will need to be rewritten to account for these new cell types, because public CBBs are currently only permitted to collect and store cord blood. Therefore, CBBs' expansion into other cell types would likely require significant additional financial investment.

International Cord Blood Banks May Continue to Increase Their U.S. Market Share

International CBBs have expanded their operations during the past decade and have taken both U.S. and global market share away from U.S. CBBs. In Chapter Four, we introduced this trend and provided its historical context. In this chapter, we explore whether this trend is likely to continue.

Some factors limit the degree to which international CBBs could continue to expand their market share. Many foreign countries have genetically homogenous populations compared with the U.S. population, which makes it almost impossible for most countries to collect and export a full genetic range of CBUs to meet U.S. and global demand. Instead, most international CBBs focus on serving their domestic populations, which, in many cases, overlaps only slightly with the U.S. and global populations. As the U.S. public inventory of CBUs continues to expand to include more HLA types and larger units, it would be reasonable to expect U.S. imports of foreign CBUs to decline, all else held equal. A similar logic dictates that even if international CBBs build larger (yet still less diverse) inventories, they will continue to rely on imports (some of which will presumably come from the United States) to meet the demand for unusual HLA types.

Although cases persist of U.S. hospitals purchasing foreign-derived CBUs when U.S.-derived alternatives of similar size are not available, hospitals tend to appreciate the quality and short turnaround times provided by U.S. CBBs, according to some cord blood system stakeholders that we interviewed. Also, international shipping will always entail at least some additional cost and time. These stabilizing factors aside, there are some grounds for concern that international CBBs will continue to gain market share at the expense of U.S. CBBs: As one HSC transplantation expert explained, the quality and consistency of international CBBs is improving.

In other respects, however, this increase in the production, size, and quality of foreign CBBs may help U.S. CBBs by contributing to the diversity, quality, and size of the global CBU inventory. As noted earlier in this chapter, the continued viability of cord blood as an option for HSC transplantation depends in part on cord blood's market momentum relative to other sources of HSCs. The more CBUs that are available and used worldwide, the more physicians gain experience and familiarity with cord blood selection criteria and cord blood transplantation protocols, and the more suppliers produce and improve cord blood–related devices and equipment, and researchers discover ways to improve cord blood transplantation and other medical applications. By contributing to the overall attractiveness and availability of cord blood as an option for HSC transplantations, foreign CBBs help all organizations participating in the global cord blood sector.

Summary

Chapter Four identifies several trends that have caused U.S. CBBs to experience financial hardship, and the potential future developments highlighted in this chapter could either reverse or exacerbate the sector's financial hardship. The potential technological developments highlighted here—ones that could significantly improve the efficacy of cord blood HSC transplants, create new medical applications for cord blood, or create new medical applications for other cells and tissues derived from umbilical cords and placentas, stand out as the main potential developments that could dramatically improve the financial prospects of U.S. CBBs. We are unable to assess the likelihood that these technological developments will pan out, nor can we estimate when they might occur.

The greatest dangers facing the cord blood system—and CBBs in particular—include the potential for a continued fall in demand for cord blood, possibly caused in part by shifts in the relative cost and efficacy of cord blood as compared with other sources of HSCs. We note that these shifts could happen in either direction, however, as the relative cost and efficacy of cord blood could improve rather than continue to decline. Other potential developments that could reduce demand for cord blood include the possibility of further increased competition from international CBBs.

Chapter Nine. Government Intervention in the Public Cord Blood System

This chapter builds on the previous chapters by considering the social value of the public cord blood banking system and how government interventions influence its different dimensions, including TNC counts, genetic diversity, and current and future value to society. Our initial goal is to estimate the value of the cord blood banking system, accounting for present demand. Next, we assess how existing government interventions have changed the public cord blood inventory along several different dimensions, such as average or minimum TNC and genetic diversity. Finally, we assess how alternative interventions could affect the cord blood system at both the bank and the industry levels.

Public Goods and the Social Value of the Public Cord Blood Banking System

As discussed in Chapter Two, CBUs are one source for HSCs that is available to treat a set of illnesses. CBUs differ from the other HSC sources in that they must be stored. As such, a repository is necessary. Private CBBs provide services to individuals and families that feel the need to bank CBUs for personal use. For families with a pre-existing propensity for diseases or when a sibling already has an illness treated through cord blood transplantation, private CBBs can be the best option. For most families, this is not the case, which is why few pediatric HSC transplantation physicians advise private cord banking unless there is a known recipient. As discussed in Chapter Two, a system of public CBBs is needed to make high-quality, genetically diverse CBUs available to the public. Having this type of CBB system will allow individuals with illnesses treated by CBUs to have access to units that would not be available in a private system. This *public good* provides value to all individuals and relies on donations to function.

As explained in Chapters One, Four, and Seven, many public CBBs are losing money and continue operating only by using funds from donations, subsidies, and larger organizations that own them. From a private-firm perspective, the benefits of operating a public CBB may not outweigh the costs. However, banks' revenues may not fully reflect the social benefits of operating a public CBB. Public CBBs provide a quasi-public good in that some of the benefits of the system may not be captured in transactions between CBBs and transplant centers or providers. Specifically, all individuals with access to advanced health care derive an insurance benefit from the availability of the international inventory of CBUs as a potential treatment source for conditions treated using cord blood, as well as for conditions that may in the future be treated by cord blood. Since most people benefitting from the insurance value of this inventory have not paid directly to build or sustain the inventory, there is a justification for government intervention to coordinate activity and—potentially—to subsidize the collection, processing, and use of cord blood. To understand if government intervention provides positive net benefits, we must understand what both the social benefits and costs are.

In this analysis, we only focus on the costs faced by public CBBs, and ignore other cord blood system costs, such as research costs. We rely on the CBB aggregated cost estimates—described fully in Chapter Six—to proxy for social costs that we need to compare with social benefits. Thus, we aim to estimate the *social* benefits that the public CBB system provides. Specifically, we are only considering the benefits of the publicly banked units that are listed on The Registry.

We consider two sets of benefits: First, there are the *direct* benefits provided by the use of cord blood for medical treatment. These direct benefits are tied to the patients' increased life span and quality of life. Second, there are several *indirect* benefits that arise from the existence of the CBB system. Without the CBB system, CBUs could not be used as a treatment for the diseases discussed in Chapter Two. In other words, there is an insurance value to having a national inventory: In the event that someone is diagnosed with a disease that is treatable with cord blood, there is a good chance that he or she will find a unit in the inventory for use. We do not measure the indirect benefits, except to say that the direct value could be weighted by the probability that any given person would need to use the system. Thus, our value calculation underestimates the total societal value.

As technology evolves, cord blood may provide treatments for additional diseases. Having CBUs and a cord blood system—including the infrastructure, knowledge, and trained staff—available now means that they will not have to be gathered in the future. Building a CBB system in the future may be more expensive than keeping the existing structure, even if the current benefits do not outweigh the costs, given current technology and use. Furthermore, we might never know what diseases could be treated by cord blood if we do not support the infrastructure today, because ongoing research partially depends on this existing cord blood infrastructure and ongoing cord blood use.

The value of the CBB system cannot be assessed without considering its connections to other stem cell sources and uses. Cord blood's value depends in part on the value of alternative sources of HSCs, and any policies designed to strengthen the cord blood system will probably create both positive and negative spillover effects on other markets. As discussed in Chapters Two and Eight, HSCs also come from peripheral blood and bone marrow donors, and technologies for collecting, processing, and using these HSCs may be advancing more quickly than cord blood–related technologies. To the extent that some medical interventions can use HSCs from sources other than cord blood, any effort to subsidize CBUs could distort the HSC market by lowering the relative cost of cord blood, thereby raising demand for cord blood and lowering demand for other sources of HSCs. On the positive side, any policies or interventions that strengthen the cord blood system could also help to advance technological progress in processing, transplanting, and finding alternative medical uses for HSCs, which could help other parts of the stem-cell sector and the broader health system.

Direct Use Value of CBB System

Three pieces of information are required to calculate the direct use value of the CBB system. First, we need to know the demand for CBUs. The data used in Chapter Five provide this information. Second, we need to be able to quantify how much the treatment improves quality and duration of life. This is complicated by the fact that alternative treatments exist that could have been used but were not, as discussed in more detail below. Finally, we need to know the economic value of the improvements to life span and quality of life.

Cord Blood Demand

Table 9.1 shows the aggregate annual demand for U.S. domestic CBUs shipped both domestically and internationally. The average annual number of CBUs used for transplants in the United States was 1,541 between 2010 and 2016. This demand is a function of the size of the international CBB system, the prevalence of diseases already treatable by cord blood, the current technology for treating diseases using cord blood transplant, the availability of alternative treatments, and the relative effectiveness of cord blood and alternative treatments. Because there has been a growing use of multicord transplants in adult patients, we used NMDP data to estimate the number of multicord transplants. Based on the NMDP data, we know that approximately 57 percent of the units shipped were part of a multicord transplant. Thus, we reduced demand by 57 percent to estimate the number of transplants rather than the number of CBUs shipped. The size of the CBB system is important because, as the number of banked CBUs increases, the genetic diversity of the inventory and the number of higher–TNC count units should increase. Consequently, as the inventory grows, the probability that any individual is able to find a suitable match also rises.[86] These combined factors increase the probability that an individual who needs an HSC transplant will receive a cord blood transplant as opposed to seeking alternative HSC sources.

Table 9.1. Aggregate Annual CBU Demand, by Year

Year	CBUs Shipped
2010	1,263
2011	1,786
2012	1,746
2013	1,684
2014	1,533
2015	1,618
2016	1,158

SOURCE: RAND authors' calculations using NMDP data (see Chapter Three for more details on this source). Table data are adapted from Figure 5.2 in this report.

An earlier study using data from the CIBMTR estimated the five-year survival rate for individuals receiving different-quality HLA matches.[86] We followed this approach, estimating the life expectancy from each treatment under three different scenarios: Scenario 1 assumes that the relative survival risk for an additional antigen mismatch is the same for cord blood and bone marrow; Scenario 2 assumes that the match level for cord blood matters, although not as much for cord blood as bone marrow; and Scenario 3 assumes that survival does not depend at all on HLA match.

In Table 9.2, we present the estimated life expectancy for these three scenarios across different match criteria for adult and pediatric patients, separately.[a] The increase in estimated life expectancy relative to no treatment for cord blood ranges from six months to five years for adult patients and 13 to 23 years for pediatric patients. We used a no-transplant counterfactual to calculate increases in life expectancy since cord blood may be viewed as a safety-net technology. That is, our analysis assumes that without cord blood, the patient would not have a source for HSCs. Alternatively, one could calculate the difference in life expectancy between a transplant from an alternative HSC source that could be available in the absence of cord blood, but which could be a poorer match quality. This approach would require assumptions about the distribution of matches. The resulting estimates of the benefits of cord blood would likely be lower than those in our analysis. At the same time, an analysis that included estimates of the insurance value of the system, higher value-of-life estimates, or estimates of the future value of the system from additional diseases treated with cord blood would yield benefit estimates that are greater than our estimates.

To provide an upper bound, we assumed an increase in life expectancy of five and 23 years for adults and children, respectively. We calculated this increase by taking the difference in life expectancy from the treatment with cord blood and no treatment using Scenario 3. From Figure 5.6, we know that approximately 43 percent of all cord blood transplants are pediatric patients and 57 percent are adults. Taken together, we estimated the weighted average of the estimated life expectancy for pediatric and adult patients that can be attributed to a cord blood transplant. Following earlier studies, we assumed that the increase in one life year is valued at $100,000.[156–158]

---

[a] These life expectancies are calculated using Howard et al. estimates for five-year survival based on data from the CIBMTR. The authors additionally assumed that if individuals do not survive to five years that they die at six months from treatment. If the individuals survive to five years, it is assumed that they live for 25 years and 68 years for adult and pediatric patients, respectively. Both of these assumptions are consistent with the CIBMTR data. As an example from Howard et al., the five-year survival for an adult receiving a 6/6 cord blood transplant has a 36-percent probability of living at least five years.[86] Thus, the expected life expectancy from this treatment is $(1-0.36) \times 0.5 + 0.36 \times 25$.

Table 9.2. Life Expectancy from Different Treatments

Transplant Type	Patients Aged 21 or Older			Patients Aged 20 or Younger		
	Scenario 1	Scenario 2	Scenario 3	Scenario 1	Scenario 2	Scenario 3
8/8 bone marrow	9.3	9.3	9.3	33.6	33.6	33.6
7/8 bone marrow	6.6	6.6	6.6	28.2	28.2	28.2
6/6 cord blood	9.3	9.3	9.3	33.6	33.6	33.6
5/6 cord blood	6.6	8.3	9.3	28.2	30.2	33.6
4/6 cord blood	4.7	7.6	9.3	23.5	27.5	33.6
No transplant	4.2	4.2	4.2	10.6	10.6	10.6

SOURCE: RAND authors' calculations based on methodology from Table 3 in Howard et al.[86]
NOTE: Scenario 1 assumes that the risk associated with HLA mismatch is the same for cord blood as it is for bone marrow with age categories; Scenario 2 assumes that HLA match matters less for cord blood than for bone marrow; and Scenario 3 assumes that there is no difference in survivability with HLA mismatch.

Use Value of the Cord Blood Bank System

Because we do not know the distribution of HLA mismatch, we use the three scenarios from Table 9.2 and then assume three different levels of matching to provide a range of potential annual values. To provide a lower bound, we used Scenario 1 and assumed that all patients received a 4/6 match. Next, as an intermediate set of assumptions, we assumed that all patients received a 5/6 match and used Scenario 2 in terms of effectiveness. Finally, we used Scenario 3 and assumed 6/6 matches to provide an upper bound. For the upper-bound estimate, we multiplied the number of annual pediatric recipients by 23 years (from Table 9.2, Scenario 3 with a 6/6 match), and for adult patients we multiplied the total adult units shipped by five years (from Table 9.2, Scenario 3 with a 6/6 match). This gives us an estimate for the *total number of life years saved over all patients who received a cord blood transplant in one year*. Finally, we multiplied total expected life years gained by $100,000 to estimate the total use value per year for the years 2010–2016. Column three in Table 9.3 displays the results. Thus, our estimates of the average annual value of the CBB system range from a lower bound of $883 million to $1.7 billion.

Table 9.3. Average Annual Social Value of the CBB System

Year	Scenario 1 4/6 Match	Scenario 2 5/6 Match	Scenario 3 6/6 Match
2010	$724,014,750	$1,374,144,000	$1,429,084,500
2011	$1,023,824,500	$1,943,168,000	$2,020,859,000
2012	$1,000,894,500	$1,899,648,000	$1,975,599,000
2013	$965,353,000	$1,832,192,000	$1,905,446,000
2014	$878,792,250	$1,667,904,000	$1,734,589,500
2015	$927,518,500	$1,760,384,000	$1,830,767,000
2016	$663,823,500	$1,259,904,000	$1,310,277,000
Annual value	$883,460,143	$1,676,763,429	$1,743,803,143

SOURCE: RAND authors' calculations.

With technological change in both cord blood and alternative stem cell therapies, the use value may increase or decrease. Importantly, changes in the value will be driven by the demand for CBUs.

Limitations of the Estimates of the Value of the Public CBB System

In addition to the direct use value estimated above, the public CBB system has value independent of current use. For instance, having a functioning CBB system means that, in the future, if technological change increases demand for cord blood, we will not have to build the system from scratch. Also, there exist at least some additional CBU sales outside of the NMDP, which increases the current use of cord blood beyond what our calculations suggest. For example, some CBUs have been sold to a biotechnology company that turns CBUs into non-HLA supplements used in cord blood transplants, increasing their efficacy. These factors increase the value of the CBB system beyond the use value that we have calculated.

Conversely, considering additional factors could decrease the value of our estimates. For example, if the CBB system did not exist, at least some patients would be forced to use alternative sources of HSCs—including CBUs from banks located in foreign countries. This ability to use a substitute technology decreases the value of the U.S. cord blood system: If cord blood were not produced in the United States, the next-best alternative HSC source would sometimes be used. Our use value calculations assume that there is no next-best alternative. Thus, the actual value may be lower when we consider alternative sources of treatment.

Our analysis is sensitive to our assumptions of costs and benefits; therefore, if we assumed greater gains in life expectancy or value of life, our estimates would be higher.

Aggregate Costs of the Cord Blood Banking Industry

An analysis by the NMDP suggests that the aggregate annual costs to the cord blood industry for recruitment, processing, and storage are on the order of $60–70 million. Even assuming the existence of additional costs for running the NMDP, for distribution to hospitals, and for research, *the social benefit of having a cord blood system far outweighs its costs*, by at least one order of magnitude. However, many of the social benefits accrue to people who have not yet paid into the system (because they do not yet need cord blood), and current users of the system do not appear willing to pay for the full societal benefit. The question then becomes how to sustain the CBB system until the point in time when cord blood demand and/or willingness to pay increases.

Objectives of the National Cord Blood Inventory Program

As stated in Chapter Two, the aim of the Stem Cell Therapeutic and Research Act is to make at least 150,000 high-quality units from a genetically diverse population available for transplant.[45] Although the legislation does not define *high-quality*, HRSA provides definitions through contracts with CBBs under NCBI. There are two main considerations for quality. First, the CBU must be collected in an appropriate manner so as to minimize risk to the transplant patient. This includes testing for infectious disease and sterility. From our perspective, these attributes of quality are embodied within the accreditation process. As HRSA requires that all NCBI CBBs must be accredited by either the AABB or the FACT, this aspect of quality should be achieved automatically.

The second aspect of quality considered by HRSA is the minimum TNC count needed for inclusion in the NCBI registry. TNC count is important because the current dosing requirements are for 2.5×10^7 TNC per kg.[159] The current HRSA minimum total TNC level corresponds to a CBU adequate for patients weighing 36 kg or less (about 80 pounds) and inadequate for the average adult in the United States. As discussed in Chapter Seven, HRSA's minimum is one of the lowest among all international CBB systems.

The other objective for HRSA is to have a unit available to everyone who needs it. This means that there must be enough genetic diversity in the NCBI program to match that of the population. The key markers for genetic diversity for HRSA are race and ethnicity. Figure 9.1 displays the racial and ethnic diversity of the banked units from 2002 to 2016 and of the U.S. population as of 2015. For 13 percent of the banked units, we do not have any data on race or ethnicity, or they are multiracial. If we assume that all the units that are labeled "other" are actually Caucasian units, then there is an over-representation of Caucasians. Alternatively, if the "other" category is equally representative of the non-Caucasian categories, the racial diversity of the banked units is approximately equal to that of the population.

From previous Requests for Proposals[b] that HRSA issued for contractor CBBs, there is a special emphasis on collecting units of African ancestry.[160] There are potentially two reasons for this emphasis. First, there may be concern that The Registry (currently or historically) has fewer African ancestry units relative to the population. It is difficult to assess this, given data limitations, but in Figure 9.1 we show that the relative proportion of banked CBUs of African ancestry is roughly in line with the population. Second, according to one expert we interviewed, the genetic diversity of African ancestry is greater than that for other ethnic groups. As such, patients of African ancestry are less likely to find a match among CBUs from other racial and ethnic groups. Thus, HRSA may strive to have an over-representation of those racial and ethnic groups that have greater genetic diversity, which is consistent with their emphasis on obtaining units from individuals of African ancestry.

Figure 9.1. Racial and Ethnic Diversity of the National Cord Blood Inventory and the U.S. Population

Racial and Ethnic Diversity of Banked Units, 2002–2016	Racial and Ethnic Diversity of U.S. Population, 2015

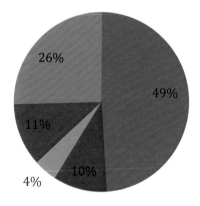 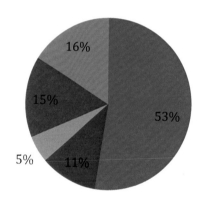

■ Caucasian ■ African American ■ Asia-Pacific Islander ■ Hispanic ■ Other

SOURCE: RAND authors' calculations using NMDP data on newly banked CBUs from 2002 to 2016. U.S. Population statistics from the U.S. Census, Quick Facts United States.

Existing Program

At present, there are 13 CBBs that are participating in the NCBI program. There have been five separate cohorts of CBBs added to the program. Although they are part of the NCBI

---

[b] Specifically, the Request for Proposals states, "special consideration will be given to offerors demonstrating a superior ability to collect and bank large numbers of CBU[s] from underrepresented populations, especially African-Americans."

program, banks are not guaranteed funding every year. In 2011, CBBs collected CBUs at 114 hospitals in 24 states for the NCBI. Additionally, there are six other CBBs that do not participate in the NCBI but list their units on The Registry. We were unable to acquire the individual contracts the CBBs have with HRSA, but a GAO report from 2011 estimates that the average subsidy paid per CBU in the NCBI was $1,110.[1]

Based on our interviews with representatives from HRSA, these subsidies are CBB-specific as delineated in a given CBB's proposal to HRSA and at least one CBB received differential payments based on race/ethnicity of the donor. HRSA representatives also stated that when they are considering contracts with CBBs, their goal is to maximize the number of units registered, given budget constraints. Because CBBs all bid different subsidy amounts, there is implicitly competition among the CBBs to bid the lowest dollar amount for HRSA to subsidize each unit. CBBs that are more financially sound may, therefore, be more willing and able to accept a smaller subsidy. If less established, less financially sound, or savvy CBBs want to compete, they too may feel the need to lower their subsidy bids, which may result in greater losses and less financial sustainability. The recent concerns about CBBs' financial sustainability may be driven in part by the subsidy and contract structures and not simply as a function of the nature of the industry.

To some extent, this situation results from payers' unwillingness to pay more for CBUs of varying sizes and HLA types. As noted earlier, CBBs charge the same fee per CBU regardless of size and HLA type, so there is a strong financial incentive for CBBs to bank only the CBUs with the highest probability of use. If, for example, CBBs were able to charge more for a rare HLA-typed unit or for a larger CBU, the market would incentivize the collection of rarer CBUs. There is already some market incentive to bank larger units versus smaller ones, because hospitals are more likely to procure larger units, but this market incentive is weaker when it comes to HLA type. Because market incentives to bank diverse units are weak, HRSA subsidies may provide additional incentives to bank rarer units. The HRSA subsidy increases the revenue CBBs receive when collecting and when distributing cord blood from ethnically diverse donors, which at least partially compensates for the lower probability that such units will be used. This does not necessarily maximize the number of lives saved by cord blood, because the money used to save some number of rare HLA-type patients may have been enough money to save twice as many common HLA-type patients. However, it does achieve the social objective of helping to level the access to cord blood across all Americans, which is the aim of the legislation and NCBI.

Potential Alternative Programs

There are a number alternative program designs that could be considered by HRSA. One option would be for HRSA to provide only a subsidy to those units that have high TNC counts or those from African and Asian/Pacific Islander ancestry. Alternatively, HRSA could subsidize units that are collected or used or provide a fixed subsidy independent of the number of units collected, banked, or shipped. We discuss each of these three possibilities in turn. Table 9.4 provides an overview of the advantages and disadvantages of each alternative subsidy arrangement.

Table 9.4. Advantages and Disadvantages of Alternative Subsidy Arrangements

Subsidy	Advantages	Disadvantages
Collected	• Encourages greater effort into collection. • Potential for greater diversity.	• Lack of verification. • May encourage higher TNC cutoff. • May reduce diversity.
Shipped	• Alignment of incentives to bank for sustainability. • Encourages greater collection efforts to obtain higher–TNC count units.	• May encourage higher TNC cutoff. • May reduce diversity if shipments to minorities are not subsidized at a higher rate. • Cost per unit banked may rise to reach higher TNC cutoff.
Lump sum	• May encourage diversity through adding hospitals with high minority birth rates. • Allows greater flexibility by CBBs to achieve financial sustainability.	• Potential lack of accountability. • Is not directly aligned with HRSA goals.

Subsidize Based on the Number of Units Collected

Suppose that HRSA were to redesign its program to subsidize not future banking, but total (previous) collection of CBUs. This would focus on the stock of CBUs—rather than the flow—and could provide additional incentive to collect more units. All else equal, this could cause more units to be banked than if no subsidy existed, because more units would be collected and more units should meet the CBB (or HRSA) TNC cutoff. Suppose we were to consider a budget-neutral program that subsidized collection instead of banking. If a CBB had a typical discard rate of 75 percent, a subsidy equal to one-fourth the size of the current subsidy for banking would have the same effect in expectation on units banked. Additionally, by focusing on collection rather than banking, the CBB has more certainty over its subsidies since it is not dependent on the TNC, which is somewhat of a random draw.

There are several potential problems with this alternative subsidy arrangement, however. First, the current system provides verification through the NMDP that the unit exists and was registered. With a collection-based subsidy, there is no built-in verification process; in other words, HRSA would be relying on the CBBs' reports of units collected. Second, there may be an incentive to further increase the TNC cutoff since the probability that a unit will be chosen for transplantation increases with higher TNC counts, so the discard rate might increase. The incentives from the subsidy would affect the number of units collected, but because CBBs tend to lose money on lower–TNC count units (as discussed in Chapter Seven), banks may choose to increase their internal TNC threshold as higher–TNC units have a higher release rate. This could translate into fewer units being added to The Registry, although they would be of higher quality.

Subsidize Based on the Number of Units Shipped for Transplantation

As another alternative, suppose that HRSA provided a subsidy only for those units that were shipped for transplantation. Since the probability of a unit being chosen increases as TNC increases, this would further encourage CBBs to raise their internal TNC thresholds for banking. Also, to collect higher-TNC units, CBBs may collect more units. With this approach, in contrast to subsidizing unit collection, verification of number of units shipped is relatively straightforward: HRSA could verify the shipment of these units through NMDP records on shipped CBUs. Importantly, by subsidizing the shipment of units, HRSA would be providing an incentive that aligns with the CBB goal of financial sustainability. We know from Table 7.2 in Chapter Seven that the higher the TNC, the higher the expected revenues from an individual banked unit. However, some might argue that HRSA should not be subsidizing something the CBBs already have an incentive to do and are already paid to do. If HRSA wanted to increase the probability that CBBs would bank units that will be shipped, they could simply increase the minimum TNC required to be subsidized. In other words, as TNC rises, profitability of the unit rises. However, the cost per unit may also rise: More units will have to be collected to find a unit that meets the higher TNC threshold.

Provide a Lump-Sum Subsidy

Finally, HRSA could provide a lump-sum subsidy for participation in the program. This lump-sum subsidy could include contingencies, such as expanding to an additional hospital that participates in collection with the CBB (e.g., with a high rate of minority births). Additionally, allowing CBBs greater flexibility in how and where they collect units may increase the financial sustainability of the CBBs. Not being tied to specific TNC cutoffs and having the ability to experiment without fear of bankruptcy may provide new approaches for collection, banking, and shipment that had not been considered before due to financial constraints.

At least one of the current CBB's contracts has differential subsidies for minority CBUs. HRSA should consider requiring this more broadly across other contracts if the social value of minority units is higher or if the social cost of collection is higher. The social value may be higher if there exists greater genetic diversity in the minority population, such that increasing the number of minority units results in better coverage of the genetic space. We also know from interviews that it is costlier to recruit minorities, both for bone marrow donation and for CBUs. We also noted earlier in the report that minority CBUs tend to be smaller in TNC count due to underlying biological differences.

From the banks' perspective, there is a trade-off between banking a lot of units and having higher, on average, TNC counts. As a bank increases the TNC cutoff, the cost per banked unit increases because more units will be discarded after collection. From HRSA's perspective, one of the main goals is genetic diversity, which requires a large number of units from a variety of races and ethnicities. From a transplant perspective, there is a trade-off between HLA-matching and TNC count. Particularly, the greater the HLA mismatch, the greater the TNC count needs to be to produce the same outcomes as a closer match. This implies that as the TNC count increases for a unit, the greater the number of potential transplants. Put differently, as the TNC count increases, fewer units are needed to achieve the same coverage in terms of genetic diversity. The goal from society's perspective should be to have a unit available to treat everyone that may need it. This can be accomplished by having a large number of units that, on average, have a low TNC count or having a smaller inventory size with units with a higher TNC count. Importantly, as average TNC increases, the cost per unit increases, but fewer units are required.

Summary

In this chapter, we estimated the value of the CBB system to be between $600 million and $2 billion annually based on increased life expectancy for patients receiving CBU transplants. Even by our most-conservative estimates of the efficacy of cord blood, the benefits of the system far outweigh the collection, processing, and storage costs of approximately $60–70 million. This suggests that there may be a larger role for government intervention to maintain this valuable resource.

The aim of the NCBI program administered by HRSA is to ensure that everyone who needs a CBU can find a match. There are two aspects that capture this: diversity and usability. The current system provides subsidies to CBUs with a minimum TNC count of 0.90×10^9, but these subsidies vary by CBB. This minimum TNC count combined with accreditation should ensure that every CBU in NCBI is usable. To encourage diversity, as part of its request for proposals from CBBs, HRSA states that special consideration will be given to proposals that put a focus on donors of African ancestry and other underrepresented groups. The distribution of donor race of CBUs appears to roughly mirror the racial distribution of the U.S. population.

Finally, we provided an analysis of alternative subsidy structures. From a transplant perspective, there is a trade-off between HLA mismatch and TNC count. There may be advantages in moving to a system that, at least partially, provides lump-sum subsidies to encourage CBBs to seek FDA licensure or to develop relationships with hospitals with larger underrepresented deliveries that may be costlier to collect.

Chapter Ten. Themes, Recommendations, and Conclusion

In this final chapter, we highlight the key findings from our study that drive the basis for the recommendations we propose to improve the sustainability of the public cord blood system. We also discuss the limitations of our study, recommendations, caveats, and areas that warrant further research.

Key Themes

Below we highlight our synthesis of themes identified across the report from more than one source.

Demand for Cord Blood Has Stagnated

Particularly, key stakeholders and our analysis of NMDP data suggests that U.S. demand for cord blood has declined or plateaued for the time being. The number of cord blood transplants performed in the United States fell slightly from 822 to 718 from 2010 to 2015.[a] Over the same period, the number of haploidentical transplants increased from 361 to 1,045, as have HSC transplants overall. Thus, cord blood transplants fell from about 12 percent of all HSC transplants to about 8 percent from 2010 to 2015.

Several explanations for this trend have been identified. In addition to occasional availability of cheaper alternatives, such as haploidentical HSCs, some have argued that CBU collection costs have increased over time as CBBs have endeavored to procure more-diverse units. These rising costs could be one factor dampening demand. Several banks noted the high cost of obtaining FDA licensure, which they state has exacerbated cord blood's cost disadvantage relative to other sources of HSCs that do not bear similar costs for compliance. Many respondents noted that delayed umbilical cord clamping may also contribute to higher collection costs, which in turn can decrease demand.

Competition Among CBBs Has Increased

The international CBB industry has matured over time, so a greater number of domestic and international CBBs are competing to provide CBUs to patients. Meanwhile, the number of U.S. CBBs and their inventory of CBUs both continue to grow. If the number of CBBs and CBUs rises while demand for cord blood remains stagnant or falls, CBBs will face financial pressure unless they can get more money per CBU shipped.

---

[a] As noted in Chapter Three, we have NMDP data on transplants for only part of 2016, so we focus on 2015 in this report. There were only 289 cord blood transplants and 4,006 total HSC transplants in the 2016 data we received.

CBB organizational and ownership structures affect their financial viability. CBBs that have survived and thrived tend to be part of larger organizations, such as blood banks, hospitals, universities, biotechnology firms, or private-public hybrid banks. These organizational strategies are significant because they allow CBBs to diversify their sources of income and make it easier for CBBs to cut costs. For example, CBBs that are connected to blood banks typically rely on some of the same infrastructure and processes used by the whole blood bank. CBBs that are affiliated with hospitals may have easier access to local labor and delivery wards, which can reduce collection costs. CBBs that are part of a university, typically in conjunction with a university hospital, are often linked to HSC-expert physicians and researchers who are more likely to be involved in clinical trials and clinical practice involving CBUs. Hybrid CBBs that do both public and private banking can achieve greater efficiencies of scale, and profits from their private operations can subsidize their public operations.

Cord Blood Procurement Costs Have Increased Relative to Alternative Sources of HSCs

We noted this above, in explaining the trends away from CBUs, but also note this separately because there are several key drivers of cost that are worth highlighting.

First, two important features of CBUs that drive costs are the TNC count and donor diversity. Obtaining higher–TNC count units increases acquisition costs because CBBs have to collect more units to get a useable or bankable "high–" TNC count unit. The actual marginal cost of collecting one extra unit does not vary by TNC count. However, costs to collect CBUs from racial minorities have been reported to be higher.

Additionally, the process of predicting the size of a CBU prior to collection is inexact. Although it is known that TNC count is positively correlated with factors such as gestational age, Cesarean delivery, and the infant's birth weight, and negatively correlated with the number of children a woman has previously given birth to, these are not one-to-one correlations. Further, some of these factors are unknown until delivery.[80] Thus, we can think of TNC count as conditionally random and therefore difficult for CBBs to target perfectly.

Although some have argued that cord blood acquisition costs are significantly higher than other sources of HSCs, we were unable to examine this empirically due to lack of data. Our analysis, however, of the HCUP data on inpatient stays suggests that the variable costs, which have been estimated to be between $1,700 and $3,100 per CBU (see Chapter Six), pale in comparison to other costs associated with HSC treatment, which are between approximately $160,000 and $262,000 per inpatient treatment (see Table 6.2). This is largely because inpatient HSC transplants typically require hospitalization, with cord blood patients requiring about 50 days of inpatient stay relative to about 38 days for allogeneic bone marrow transplant patients. We also point out that the calculation of costs associated with bone marrow or other peripheral stem cell sources typically does not include costs to the donor, except to note that it often takes more time to obtain HSCs from these sources. A consideration of the actual health care costs of collecting the bone marrow or other HSCs, the preparation and time required of the donor, and the physical pain should be factored into these comparisons. Any comparison of costs, however, should be accompanied by a comparison of benefits and the importance of diversifying stem cell sources, particularly for patients for whom a bone marrow or peripheral blood match is not readily available.

The Relative Clinical Effectiveness of Cord Blood Transplantations Versus Other HSC Transplantations Remains Unclear in Some Medical Scenarios

Existing studies on the effectiveness of the different HSC sources (see Chapter Six) are problematic for several reasons. First, comparison of patients across the different HSC sources is difficult because selection of an HSC source is clearly not random. Some of our key interviewees shared that CBUs are used only as a last resort, whereas others mentioned a preference for CBUs, particularly for certain types of patients. Thus, any comparison of patients using different HSC sources suffers from a significant selection bias. This can be addressed, somewhat, in randomized controlled trials, but in such a study, the sample will have to be restricted to patients for whom all sources are available, which limits the generalizability of findings.

Second, the majority of the literature to date on clinical effectiveness follows patients for only a short time period. Because cord blood transplants take longer to engraft, such a time frame truncation will bias results toward more-favorable outcomes for other sources. For example, a 2007 systematic review shows the average survival of cord blood transplant patients at 47 percent (95-percent confidence interval [CI] = 38.6 percent, 55 percent) within the first 100 days relative to 62 percent (95-percent CI = 57 percent, 68 percent) for bone marrow or other peripheral blood stem cell transplants. However, at five years out, survival rates were 14.4 percent (95-percent CI = 10 percent, 18.8 percent) and 18.2 percent (95-percent CI = 13.8 percent, 22.6 percent) for cord blood and other HSC transplant patients, respectively, suggesting no statistically significant difference. There are considerably fewer studies examining longer-term survival rates in this review. Finally, it is worth pointing out that even if CBUs yield better patient outcomes over the longer term, payer reimbursement preferences may render this moot. Specifically, because patients tend to change health insurance plans or coverage every few years, private insurers prefer to cover services that are less expensive in the short-to-medium term.

Cord Blood Transplantation Is Not a Panacea Treatment, but Its Availability Is Important

CBUs are one important tool among many for the treatment of some diseases. CBUs are not the answer for every patient needing a bone marrow transplant, but their availability is crucial for hundreds of patients every year who have no alternative treatment modality. Particularly, cord blood transplants can be critical for pediatric and minority populations. Although sometimes there are alternatives to cord blood, patients often have no appropriate alternative HSC source. In addition, the importance of getting treatment quickly for some patients can make CBUs the best choice compared with other HSC sources that require greater lead time. It can take two or more weeks to obtain other sources of HSCs, whereas already-banked CBUs can be ready in a fraction of that time.

Several key interviewees noted that, at the current time, if cord blood were to disappear as a treatment option it would result in increased mortality, particularly for minority populations who depend on the diversity conferred by cord blood and for pediatric populations, who are not only more diverse compared with adult populations but are generally smaller than adult patients and may therefore be treated using some of the smaller CBUs in the inventory. Thus, despite its relatively infrequent use, there is an argument to be made for supporting the cord blood industry for the sake of equity.

There Is Considerable (Positive and Negative) Uncertainty About the Future Use of Cord Blood

Changes in technology or new research findings related to the use of HSCs might dramatically increase or decrease the future use of cord blood. Clinical trials experimenting with cord blood use typically address rare diseases, but some respondents mentioned cord blood as a source for CAR T-cells, and they mentioned research into new cord blood applications to treat diabetes, traumatic brain injury, stroke, cerebral palsy, and autism. Any new medical applications for cord blood could dramatically increase demand for CBUs. There is also promising research on HSC expansion and related technologies that could increase the utility of small CBUs. The impact of expansion technologies is unclear: It might boost demand for CBUs and help some of the low–TNC count CBUs be utilized. However, in the long run, depending on the degree to which expansion technologies are effective, they might eliminate the need for new cord blood collections if transplant centers or CBBs could maintain a "library" of diverse CBUs that could be expanded at will. Furthermore, if new medical applications for cord blood do not pan out, or if other sources of HSCs prove equally able to provide the same medical benefits for a lower price, future demand for cord blood could stagnate or decline.

Recommendations

We have identified several areas in the cord blood industry where policies could plausibly improve the financial sustainability of the U.S. public cord blood system.

Our first set of recommendations pertains to the NCBI program. We have described the attributes of the current NCBI program as administered by HRSA earlier in this report. Briefly, HRSA currently provides subsidies to contractor banks that register CBUs with a minimum TNC count of 0.9×10^9 with a stated goal of increasing the racial and ethnic diversity of the units in the inventory. We begin by discussing recommendations for potentially adjusting this program, both with respect to the TNC threshold and how subsidies are structured. We then discuss some potential adjustments to NCBI contracts.

Our second set of recommendations includes broader suggestions for the industry, including suggestions for revisions to payment for cord blood transplants, research funding, and knowledge-sharing in the industry.

Recommendations for the NCBI Program

Subsidies and CBU Requirements

TNC Threshold. Our economic analysis in Chapter Seven suggests that, on average, even with the NCBI subsidies, CBBs lose money for every unit collected that has a TNC count of less than 1.5×10^9. Moreover, a CBU with a total TNC count between 0.9 and 1.24×10^9 will be used only in about one-tenth of one percent (0.1 percent) of cord blood transplants in a given year. Currently, there are over 102,000 CBUs containing less than 1.25×10^9 cells, including non-NCBI units, listed on The Registry (about 52 percent).

Current research indicates that a higher TNC count can offset some degree of HLA mismatch. Thus, if one of HRSA's objectives is to increase ethnic and racial minorities' access to cord blood, it can accomplish this by incentivizing CBBs to collect higher–TNC count units. Some stakeholders have previously recommended this threshold be increased to 1.25×10^9 for minority units and 1.5×10^9 for nonminority units.[135] Although HRSA representatives have emphasized that their current minimum does not preclude banks from setting their own higher threshold if it makes business sense for an individual bank, we emphasize that the current structure incentivizes CBBs to bank smaller units to receive the NCBI subsidy. Although banks lose money in the long term, banking smaller units to collect the NCBI subsidy helps with short-term cash flow.

These banks are also partially motivated by altruism. If a CBB's management is willing to take a financial loss to help address a need for rare HLA types, the NCBI subsidy defraying even part of that financial loss could be the deciding factor that convinces CBBs to do what is not in their long-term financial interest. To date, 47 percent of the NCBI units banked have TNC counts of less than 1.25×10^9. Given the 0.1-percent chance that units with less than 1.25×10^9 cells will be used, increasing the inventory of low–TNC count units does not translate into greater access for minorities, as long as cell expansion technologies remain under development.

The significant downside of increasing the minimum threshold is that doing so will result in fewer units added to the national inventory, which may have implications for improving the genetic diversity of the inventory (see Chapter Seven). However, given the growth in the inventory since the beginning of the NCBI program, focusing on the collection of higher–TNC count units, especially nonminority units, would be the strategy most likely to further improve access to the system. On the other hand, if future cell expansion technologies, some of which are currently under development, succeed in expanding smaller units into bigger units, a small but genetically diverse inventory may prove valuable, and the current NCBI incentives may eventually prove optimal for maximizing access. Either way, because changing the minimum threshold has implications for the genetic diversity of the inventory, we consider this in conjunction with a second related aspect of the NCBI program that could be revamped: the subsidies.

Subsidies. Currently, CBBs that are NCBI contractors propose various structures that will result in an NCBI subsidy for each CBU that is banked and listed on The Registry that meets HRSA's TNC-count threshold and other requirements. Some banks receive the subsidy only for banking minority units, while others receive the subsidy only for CBUs of a certain size. Although this gives CBBs flexibility to propose a variety of arrangements, HRSA could revise the requirements of such arrangements as outlined in Chapter Nine to achieve different goals. We review some options in the sections below.

Subsidize Based on the Number of Units Collected Instead of Units Banked or Registered on The Registry

Overall, we expect subsidies based on units collected to result in more units collected. However, the effect this would have on the average quality or TNC count of the units in the national inventory is unclear. Although some CBBs have already established internal TNC thresholds that are greater than 0.9 billion, we know that other banks continue to bank a large percentage (as much as 60 percent of all NCBI units banked) of these lower–TNC count units. As long as the revenue from the subsidy does not exceed the cost of banking an additional unit— as is currently the case—CBBs will have an incentive to try to bank units with a high probability of being used. Predicting whether a given pregnancy will yield a high–TNC count CBU is not an exact science. However, there may be room for some CBBs that are currently collecting and banking a significant percentage of low–TNC count CBUs to better screen mothers prior to delivery to increase the TNC counts of their collected units. The advantage of this approach is that a greater number of collections provides greater opportunities for collecting high–TNC count units. A disadvantage is that most public CBBs rely on hospital volunteer collectors to collect cord blood. Therefore, it is unclear what leverage or capacity CBBs may have to increase the rate of collections. In addition, the effect on minority collections may be minimal.

Subsidize Based on the Number of Units Sold for Transplant

This option could encourage CBBs to alter their collection practices, including diversity and TNC counts, to collect units that are more likely to be used. The advantage of this approach is that this arrangement would align CBBs' financial needs with the need to collect units with a high probability of being used. Thus, it might incentivize CBBs to collect larger TNC units. The disadvantage is that most transplant recipients are Caucasian; thus, the units most likely to be used are those from Caucasian donors, although this disadvantage could be overcome if NCBI provided higher subsidies for CBUs transplanted to minority patients. More concerning is that some factors associated with high TNC counts are not predictable and there may be more than one HSC match for any given patient, so it is difficult for CBBs to target high–TNC count

CBUs. Finally, this approach may be less palatable to policymakers because, in effect, CBBs would receive subsidies for the units that banks already have an incentive to collect. However, if policymakers agree that supporting the CBBs most attuned to the needs of patients is the best way to ensure continued access to cord blood, subsidizing CBB sales may work. Especially if the overall financial viability of U.S. CBBs continues to decline, with the accompanying danger of many CBBs closing, saving the strongest among these CBBs could become the priority mechanism for ensuring continued access to cord blood.

In addition to increasing the likelihood that banked CBUs correlate more closely with use, two options address the banking of minority units. Our analysis suggests that, although the current arrangement has achieved one goal of increasing the CBU inventory, it has not sufficiently incentivized the other goal of collecting high–TNC count or genetically diverse units. Particularly, if market mechanisms were working, we would expect banks to choose to bank higher–TNC count units primarily because these units are the most profitable—high–TNC count units are the most likely to be used in transplants, thus generating the greatest revenues for CBBs. In the current system, NCBI banks are encouraged to bank or register as many units (above the 0.9×10^9-TNC-count threshold) as possible with the government providing no incentive to focus on whether the units will be used. There is also no direct incentive for banks to increase the genetic diversity of CBUs: HRSA encourages banks to target minorities, and some CBBs include this in their NCBI contracts. However, there is no systematic approach to require banks to have a collection plan or strategy to increase minority units. We present two options for doing so below.

Implement Differential Subsidies for Units Banked Based on the TNC Count and/or the Genetic Diversity of the Units

Because CBBs have noted that collection costs are greater for higher–TNC count and minority units, HRSA could explicitly address this by requesting that CBBs propose this in their bids. As we have noted, some banks do this already, but a more systematic approach could optimize the collection of larger and more-diverse CBUs. This option could incentivize additional collection of units with higher TNC counts and/or more-diverse units. One disadvantage is that banks would likely incur increased costs to collect these units.

Provide Lump-Sum Subsidies to Encourage Collection of Minority Units

HRSA might consider lump-sum subsidies to offset the fixed costs associated with expanding to a new collection site or implementing some other approach to increase the collection of minority units. For example, a CBB may be interested in adding a new collection site at a hospital with a high percentage of minority births, and such a subsidy would help with the start-up and fixed costs of implementing such a move. These subsidies could also be used in efforts to recruit minority donors at existing collection sites. The advantage of this option is that it may allow for more-targeted approaches to increase the genetic diversity of the national inventory. The disadvantage is that such an approach may be more expensive than the current program.

Make Donation a Default Option

Using behavioral economics coupled with lump-sum funding to create "nudges" is one promising strategy to increase cord blood donations. *Nudges* are modest adjustments to the environment that influence "people's behavior in a predictable way without forbidding any options or significantly changing their economic incentives."[161] Examples include establishing a specific course of action as the default, framing information to emphasize risks or benefits, asking individuals to justify a planned course of action, and comparing individuals with their peers. Currently, potential parents must actively elect to donate cord blood following a birth. Changing the default option such that parents at public CBB collection hospitals who do *not* wish to donate their baby's cord blood must actively opt out of donation would likely increase the volume and diversity of cord blood cells donated to CBBs. Similar changes in the default option have led to sizable increases in organ donations.[162] Further, because umbilical cord blood is typically discarded as medical waste if it is not donated, changing the default option to cord blood donation does not harm patients.

In Table 10.1, we present a matrix that shows our hypotheses for how the market might respond depending on the set of joint changes HRSA might make for the minimum TNC-count threshold (no change or increase) and various changes to subsidy arrangements.

Thus, our recommendation is that HRSA **focus on efforts to increase the diversity of the national inventory** in the following ways: (1) provide funding that encourages banks to either add collection sites where more minority CBUs can be collected or increase subsidies for minority units, and (2) consider increasing the minimum TNC-count threshold, especially for nonminority units. HRSA might also explore ways in which CBBs might specialize in the collection of different types of units. For example, since the cost of collecting more minority units may be lower in areas with denser minority populations, CBBs with collection hospitals in these areas might specialize in collecting CBUs from minority populations, while CBBs with predominantly Caucasian populations at their collection hospitals might focus on collecting large units, which are often easier to obtain from Caucasian patients. Although we were unable to investigate this question empirically, future research may be encouraged in this area to help rationalize collection strategies.

Table 10.1. Potential Changes to the NCBI Program and Expected Effects

Changes to Subsidy Arrangements	Changes to TNC-Count Minimum Threshold	
	None	**Increase**
None	Status quo	Many banks that have already instituted internal thresholds that are higher than the HRSA threshold will be unaffected. Other banks may bank fewer units overall or a greater number of CBUs with higher–TNC count units. Overall, the inventory may grow less rapidly, but with an increase in the inventory of higher–TNC count units.
Subsidize units collected	More units collected. Banks will keep their incentive to collect higher–TNC count units as those are more likely to be sold. Likely little impact on minority collections.	More units collected. Higher minimum TNC count may offset concerns that CBBs would pay less attention to quality. Increased TNC threshold may occur naturally when banks no longer have an incentive to keep lower-quality units.
Subsidize units sold	Incentives to bank high–TNC count units may increase. May also encourage collection of more units to find high-quality units. Likely little impact on minority collections.	More units with a higher probability of being sold could be collected; i.e., higher–TNC count units. Overall, the inventory may grow less rapidly, but with increases in the inventory of higher–TNC count units.
Subsidize minority banked units differentially	CBBs would collect more genetically diverse units.	CBBs would collect more high–TNC count minority units. However, the inventory may grow less rapidly.
Offer lump-sum subsidy for certain fixed costs	Lump sum could be used to add new collection sites serving more minorities.	CBBs would collect more high–TNC count minority units. However, the inventory may grow less rapidly.

Recommendations for General Contract Terms with NCBI Banks

We briefly highlight several potential adjustments to NCBI contracts with public CBBs that could improve the operations of the CBB market in the sections below.

Replacement of Used Units

There is currently a clause in HRSA's NCBI contracts that requires banks to replace CBUs that are used for anything other than cord blood transplants if the bank has received an NCBI subsidy for the unit. There is also the issue that many of the units that have received the NCBI subsidy are too small to be used for transplants under current market conditions. In some cases, it may be beneficial to make some of those units available for research, but this contract requirement discourages such use. Further, if a higher–TNC count threshold is instituted, these small units would no longer continue to be banked, but a significant inventory of NCBI-subsidized units that are too small to be used would remain. It may be possible to negotiate with public CBBs for some form of partial reimbursement for NCBI subsidies when these too-small units are used for research purposes.

110

Standardization of Contracts

Standardized contracts with, for example, more-explicit requirements for differential thresholds or subsidies by TNC count or for minority units across all CBUs may help streamline the contracting process and improve transparency, which may impact the sustainability of individual CBBs. Standardizing some elements of the contracts could remove some of the competition from the marketplace. Although some may advocate for letting this competition play out in the marketplace, it may come at the cost of losing CBBs that could be critical to increasing the diversity of the national inventory. As noted above, there may be room for encouraging more specialization in the collection practices of CBBs to achieve greater unit diversity. Moreover, standardizing at least some of the elements of the contracts will improve transparency in the industry, which is important for evaluating the effectiveness of the government's involvement.

Provision of Consistent Funding

Although we were unable to examine data from contracts beyond what is publicly available, we note that NCBI banks are often not funded every year. This variation in funding levels can increase uncertainty for banks and may cause year-to-year hardships. Thus, we suggest that funding be offered every year if possible to bring about predictability of revenue. This may require funding fewer CBBs. This aspect could also be incorporated into the standardization of the contracts.

FDA Licensure

FDA licensure was a common area of concern in our interviews. Our understanding is that although banks initially expected stricter enforcement for nonadherence to the requirement that NCBI banks obtain FDA licensure, there has been little enforcement to date. As of this writing, HRSA has begun prioritizing licensed CBUs with the stated preference of purchasing these units over nonlicensed units, but we were unable to examine to what extent this is happening. There were also concerns that banks that did obtain licensure were being penalized as HRSA was imposing stricter requirements on those banks (e.g., withdrawn units used must be replaced with licensed units; licensed banks can only receive NCBI subsidies for licensed units, whereas unlicensed banks can receive NCBI subsidies for IND units). Our recommendation is that **HRSA consider either subsidizing differentially for licensed units or offering lump-sum funding for CBBs to obtain FDA licensure.** This could potentially be offered retroactively for CBBs that have already obtained licensure.

Contingency Planning

More broadly, HRSA could consider ways to mitigate the downside risks of industry consolidation, which may be inevitable. For example, if a public CBB is consistently unprofitable and decides to exit the market, what happens to its inventory? Contingencies for protecting those units in case of adverse events, such as bankruptcy, should be developed.

111

Having funding to allow for emergency recovery of such units (or preservation before a new owner is found) would ensure that those units do not become unviable.

Broader Recommendations for Public Cord Blood Banking

Beyond subsidies and other payment policies, in this section we discuss several other strategies that may help ensure sustainability of the public cord blood banking industry in the United States.

Payment

One repeated suggestion in our key stakeholder interviews was that payers, particularly public payers, should reimburse HSC transplants the same way organ transplants are covered. Organ transplant centers typically track the cost of acquiring organs over the course of a year to establish a standard acquisition charge that is then billed to insurers, along with the actual costs of the inpatient stay. Many private payers already cover CBU acquisition costs separately, as well as travel and lodging costs for patients.

Payments for CBUs are typically bundled into a single payment for an inpatient hospital stay for Medicare patients, but this payment does not always fully cover the costs of acquiring the CBU itself. Medicare does use the "pass-through" payment model used for organ transplants in some settings, but such a change may not yield an immediate increase in reimbursement rates. In other words, even if CMS pays separately for CBUs, doing so would not necessarily increase the total amount reimbursed for a given DRG, at least in the short term. CIBMTR has noted that hospitals do not adequately report acquisition costs to CMS and, though allowing for a separate charge for acquisition would encourage hospitals to improve coding and cost tracking, the change to reimbursement would likely lag by at least two years.[97]

A change to Medicare payment policy allowing providers to bill separately for the acquisition of HSCs, however, may change the provider calculus in deciding which source of stem cells to use. Based on the HCUP data analysis presented in Table 6.4 in Chapter Six, providers have reported costs for allogeneic bone marrow transplants at around $114,000 versus costs for cord blood transplants at around $150,000. Although our data do not allow us to observe the drivers of that difference in reported costs, our key interviewees consistently noted the significantly greater acquisition cost for CBUs. Removing the potential burden of these greater acquisition costs may result in more providers favoring cord blood as a source of HSCs.

Knowledge-Sharing

CIBMTR already helps facilitate learning collaboratives and disseminates information regarding cord blood and other HSC transplant sources to the public, researchers, and clinicians. Funding to support such activities should continue, and might even expand to encourage more-formal channels for mentoring centers with little cord blood transplantation experience by centers with extensive experience. For instance, our key interviewees representing both public

CBBs and transplant centers noted that centers with more experience performing cord blood transplants are better at selecting the right CBU. Such knowledge could be more formally shared between high-volume and low-volume transplant centers. Data from 2014 to 2015 indicate that 21 transplant centers performed more than 20 cord blood transplants.[163] Seven centers performed more than 50 transplants. Although some degree of mentorship already occurs informally, formalizing and supporting such knowledge-sharing channels could help more transplant centers gain expertise with cord blood transplants and thereby achieve better outcomes.

Research

There is ongoing research on CBUs to expand their medical applications efficacy. However, one key interviewee, a researcher who uses cord blood, noted that in a recent National Institutes of Health study section, an application using cord blood was scored poorly because one reviewer said that cord blood was no longer being used clinically. It is important for CIBMTR and others to continue emphasizing that despite the growth of haploidentical transplants, and the fact that cord blood is used for a relatively small number of HSC transplants annually, these are patients who may have no alternative source for HSCs; therefore, the treatment is vital and life-saving.

Beyond basic research, it is important to continue supporting health services research related to cord blood. For instance, it may be worthwhile to consider studies of the potential supply-chain challenges to procuring CBUs in a timely fashion. A broader analysis of the current and future barriers to procuring HSCs in a timely manner may be warranted, especially as cord blood and other HSCs expand to be used for treatment in diabetes or rare disorders, such as encephalopathy. For example, prior to the NCBI program, timeliness was a significant concern.[164]

Summary

In this report, we endeavored to understand the economics of the cord blood industry in the United States, paying particular attention to identifying current challenges and the economic viability of the public sector as well as the extent to which government policies may improve the long-term economic sustainability of the market. Our report's main objectives were to (1) describe the existing public CBB system, (2) assess current trends and economic relationships from the perspective of key stakeholders, and (3) provide recommendations for ways to improve the system. Underlying these objectives, *cord blood system sustainability* implies that there should be enough banks in the industry financially "breaking even" to maintain the current inventory and increase the diversity and quality of the units collected in the future.

We found that the demand for CBUs has recently plateaued, while demand for other HSC sources continues to increase. Physicians consider a wide range of factors in deciding which source is best for their patients, and cord blood is not a panacea treatment, but its availability is important. For some patients, it may be the only HSC source available, and for some other patients it may be the most clinically effective source of HSCs. Although stakeholders noted that the collection of cord blood is expensive, our analysis suggests that the largest factor that explains the difference in treatment costs by HSC source is the engraftment period, because it translates into significantly longer hospital stays for cord blood patients. The evidence on the clinical effectiveness of cord blood relative to other HSC sources is inconclusive because the literature focuses primarily on short-term outcomes and tends to suffer from selection bias.

We also highlighted the ongoing tension between CBBs' financial needs and their mission to provide a public good, particularly in ensuring CBU availability for minority populations. We estimated a significant societal value to having a national cord blood inventory—at about 2.5 times the annual cost of maintaining the sector—that suggests that if the market for public CBBs does not adequately provide for that inventory, government efforts to avoid market failure would be warranted. We investigated current federal involvement in the market through HRSA's NCBI program and suggested several areas for improvement. The NCBI program has clearly been effective at increasing the national inventory of CBUs, but half of the current national inventory is made up of CBUs that have TNC counts of less than 1.25 billion cells per unit, whereas the probability that a CBU with that cell count will be used in a given year is about one-tenth of one percent (or about an 11-percent chance that it will *ever* be used). As we discuss in the report, higher–TNC count units are also more likely to improve access for minority patients because CBUs that are large enough can offset HLA mismatches in some ways. We suggested several ways in which HRSA could improve the genetic diversity of the national inventory and ways in which to improve the NCBI program more broadly. We also suggested ways in which different aspects of the industry might be strengthened by potential changes to payment, research funding, and knowledge-sharing.

Appendix A. Interview Protocols

Cord Blood Banks

Introduction

- Please describe your organization's role as it relates to umbilical cord blood units (CBUs).
- Do you typically compete with other public cord blood banks (CBBs) or private CBBs or both? To your knowledge, how do CBBs, hospitals, and providers in your health care market work together to collect and utilize CBUs?
- Over the last few years, have you noticed more CBBs entering the market or any CBBs leaving the market? Why do you think they are entering/leaving?
- What kinds of market-level statistics or metrics does your CBB monitor to inform your planning broadly or in thinking about specific challenges you are facing?

How Your CBB Works

- Tell us a little bit about your CBB size—in terms of employees, number of locations, whether the bank has other product lines, and how many CBUs you have in inventory.
- How many CBUs does your CBB collect each year? Approximately how many of these are considered "high–TNC count" (or what percentage)? How many units are from minority populations or diverse HLA (or what percentage)?
- Does your CBB also perform research? If so, please describe the research.
- How does your CBB interface with The Registry of the C. W. Bill Young Cell Transplantation Program? How are new CBUs listed with The Registry?
- Do you have contractual arrangements with hospitals/providers to provide CBUs? Or are CBUs withdrawn only by finding a match on The Registry?
- What are the main current challenges for cord blood collection and utilization?

For U.S. Food and Drug Administration–Licensed Centers Only

We understand that only a handful of CBBs have obtained the U.S. Food and Drug Administration (FDA) licensure from the Office of Cellular, Tissue, and Gene Therapies. We are interested in learning more about the process, costs, and benefits of obtaining this licensure.

- When did your CBB first obtain the license and how long did the process take from application to approval?
- Can you tell us about the FDA licensure process? What were the costs of becoming an FDA-licensed center? [*Assume we collect with specific costs and indirect costs (i.e., had to hire an additional person to track processes).*]
- Why does your CBB maintain FDA licensure? What are the benefits and drawbacks of FDA licensure?
- Does licensure impact payment? If so, how?

For Unlicensed Centers Only

We understand that only a handful of CBBs have obtained FDA licensure from the Office of Cellular, Tissue, and Gene Therapies, and the CBBs that do not have this licensure use the Investigational New Drug (IND) Application instead.

- Did your CBB consider attaining FDA licensure? Why or why not?
- Are there benefits that are not available to you because you are not FDA licensed?
- How might costs change if you were *required* to obtain FDA Biologics License Application (BLA) licensure?
- What is the process for applying for and obtaining the IND exemption? Which party (blood bank, requesting physician, transplant center, cord blood registry) most commonly requests the IND exemption, in your experience?

Recruitment and Screening

- Tell us about the process of recruitment/marketing. How do potential donors learn about your CBB? What types of information do they receive?
- Do you have a sense for why donors choose your CBB over others?
- Are potential donors screened to assess the potential quality of the CBUs *prior* to collection? If so, how is this done? Are any potential donations declined due to likelihood of low-quality CBUs?
- Does your CBB do any follow-up with the family or baby following collection to assess health status, delivery complications, or other concerns? When is this done and how is this done?
- [*If not already clear*] Are any (other) donations or deposits declined prior to collection because of low quality or other reasons? [*Potential probes: multiple gestations, prematurity, chorrioamnionitis, Premature Rupture of Membranes, tear in cord intersection from placenta, other.*]

  - Are those declined donations or deposits used for any other purpose?

Cord Blood Collection

- Tell us about the process by which your organization collects CBUs.

  - Who collects the CBUs? Staff from your CBB? Staff at hospitals?
  - What sort of training do CBU collection staff receive?
  - What special equipment is required, and do you supply it or does the hospital supply it?

- Once a CBU is collected, what testing is done? Is testing performed in your CBB or elsewhere? [*Potential probes: Hemoglobinopathies, ABO Group, Rhesus (Rh) Group, infectious disease testing, Health Questionnaires, other screening?*]

  - [*If not already clear*] What procedures or strategies does your CBB pursue to ensure that high-quality CBUs are obtained?
  - What are the most important criteria that signify a high-quality CBU in your CBB?

- Are any CBUs discarded after collection because of quality or other concerns?

116

- Are these CBUs used for any other purpose? What percentage of discarded CBUs are utilized for research?

- About how many CBUs does your CBB discard per year? [*If not already clear*] What is the threshold for discarding a CBU?
- What happens after the CBUs are collected? How are they transported to your CBB? What special handling procedures are employed?
- Tell us about your organization's processes and systems for tracking collected CBUs. Do you use any software/systems, equipment, and/or tools to manage your cord blood collection and stock? [*Probes: Excel spreadsheet, Access database, another database.*]
- How do you determine which hospitals will collect CBUs for your CBB?
- Is your bank a National Cord Blood Inventory Program Contractor? How does that affect your collection processes? Can you explain how the program works in terms of the program requirements from CBBs and funding from the program?

Cord Blood Storage and Maintenance

- Tell us what happens once collected CBUs arrive at your CBB.
- What processing takes place after CBUs arrive at the CBB for storage?

  - Whole blood? Volume reduction only? Reagent Red Cells (RRC) depleted/Mononuclear cell product? Other? If more than one method, describe what determines one storage method versus another.

- What quality checks are in place to ensure appropriate storage?
- Can you describe how your CBB codes and tracks stored CBUs?
- How closely does your CBB monitor the quality of CBUs in storage and what measures are typically used to evaluate their quality?
- Is there any testing or product check that occurs during storage?
- Do you have a central storage location or several distributed throughout the country?

CBU Withdrawal

- Tell us about the process of withdrawing a CBU from your CBB.

  - What are the requirements for withdrawing a CBU? What criteria need to be met? Who sets these standards?
  - How long is a CBU typically stored before it is withdrawn?
  - What percentage of your CBUs are used each year?
  - How often do you receive a request to withdraw a CBU? Do requests ever go unfulfilled? For what reasons?
  - Is there any testing that occurs at withdrawal? Are CBUs discarded at this point for any reason?
  - What processing is done by your CBB when it is withdrawn for use? Do different end users have different requirements for the CBUs requested?

- Describe the chain of custody of a CBU that is being withdrawn for us.

Contract Costs and Payments:

We are interested in learning about the economics of CBBs.

- What are you typically paid for one CBU? At what point in the process are you paid? (e.g., at withdrawal only is likely for public banks.)

  – What is the structure of payment arrangements between your organization and hospitals? A single payment per unit? Per-unit payment? Some combination of the two? Something else?
  – Do you receive payment from the hospital or directly from the insurance company?
  – Does the payment amount differ based on the payer? (i.e., Medicaid versus Medicare versus private insurer; one geographic location versus another.)
  – Does the payment amount differ based on its quality, HLA type, use (transplant versus research), or other factors?

- [*If not already clear*] What works well about the current arrangements with your CBU users? What problems exist? What changes would you make to the current system?
- Do you feel that your organization is adequately compensated for cord blood delivered from your CBB? Why or why not? Do you have concerns about this going forward in the future?
- Aside from revenues from a withdrawal of a CBU, what are your other sources of funding? (Include percentage of total, if known.) National Institutes of Health? Private/philanthropy? State funding? Other?

Health Care System Trends

- Are there any innovations that may change the market significantly for your CBB? [*Potential probes: regenerative medicine, cell expansion for CBUs, use of double cords, etc.*]
- What trends or developments in the health care system are you worried about or have the potential to negatively impact your business?

  – [*Probe on affordable care organizations, global payments, Affordable Care Act coverage expansion, medical device excise tax, consolidation of hospital markets, regulatory requirements.*]
  – Do you have any plans to make changes (e.g., business practices) to address these threats? If yes, please describe. What about your industry more broadly—are others making changes?

- What trends or developments in the health care system are you excited about? What trends or developments have the potential to positively impact your business?

  – [*Probe on affordable care organizations, global payments, Affordable Care Act coverage expansion, medical device excise tax, consolidation of hospital markets.*]
  – Do you have any plans to make changes (e.g., business practices) to take better advantage of these opportunities? If yes, please describe. What about your industry more broadly—are others making changes?

- We are thinking about how to improve the sustainability of the U.S. cord blood system. Do you have any concerns about the sustainability of the system as it currently exists or any recommendations to improve how cord blood is managed?

Hospitals and Transplant Centers

Introduction

- Please describe your role in the organization as it relates to umbilical CBUs.
- Please describe the market for cord blood in your geographic area. How many CBBs do you work with?
- We understand that patients typically find a match through The Registry such that you would just work with the CBB with the matched CBU. Are there ever multiple matches? If yes, how do you decide which CBU to request?
- For patients who have privately banked CBUs, do you ever forego their use to go to the public registry? In what situations is this done?
- Over the last few years, have you noticed more CBBs entering the market or any CBBs leaving the market? Why do you think they are entering or leaving? Has this affected how many transplants occur in your hospital?
- Could you tell us a little about how this organization uses CBUs? When do you use CBUs versus other modalities for treatment? For research?
- Tell us what the considerations for using cord blood are for the purposes of clinical care—specific total nucleated cell (TNC) level, etc. How do these considerations differ for research purposes?
- From your perspective, what are the risks of using CBU as a treatment modality? The benefits? What are the risks and benefits of using CBUs for research?

Demographics and Logistics

- How many CBUs does your hospital use each year?

  - How many of these CBUs are used for transplants versus research?
  - For transplants, how many are conducted in pediatric versus adult populations?
  - What percentage of CBUs for transplant are considered high TNC or high CD34? What percentage of CBUs for research are considered high TNC or high CD34?
  - How many units are from minority populations or diverse HLA lines?

- [*If relevant*] Please describe the research conducted at this hospital using CBUs.
- Can you describe the process of searching for a match and requesting the units for withdrawal?

  - Are there certain HLA types that are more difficult to find a match for? How often is no match found? What are the alternatives in those cases?

- What are the main current challenges for obtaining cord blood?

Cord Blood Collection

- Does your hospital collect any CBUs, either for your own use or for deposit or donation for public or private CBBs?

    - If so, tell us about the process of collecting CBUs at your hospital.

        - Who collects the CBUs? Does your organization have any specific policies regarding the training and/or qualifications of staff who handle CBUs? i.e., is this run by pathologists? Hematologists/Oncologists? Others?

- What are the main challenges your hospital faces with CBU donation, collection, and use?
- Once a CBU is collected at your hospital, does your hospital conduct its own testing? If so, please describe the testing. [*Potential probes: Hemoglobinopathies, ABO Group, Rh Group, infectious disease testing, Health Questionnaires, other screening?*]
- Does your hospital discard any CBUs after collection because of quality or other concerns?

    - Are these CBUs used for any other purpose?
    - About how many CBUs does your hospital discard per year? [*If not already clear*] What is the threshold for discarding a CBU?

- What happens after the CBUs are collected? How are they transported to the CBB? What special handling procedures are employed?
- Does any of this differ for units that are collected for private storage?
- Are any CBUs collected that are not donated to public CBBs or deposited in private CBBs? What happens to those CBUs?

CBU Use

- Walk us through the process, from your perspective, of obtaining a CBU for a patient who needs it. Include cost considerations, if they are a factor. Do most of your requests go through The Registry? Directly to a partner CBB? Do you ever need to go to more than one source?

    - [*If relevant*] How does this process differ if the CBU is needed for research?

- [*If not already clear*] What are the requirements for withdrawing a CBU? What criteria need to be met? Who sets these standards?

    - Do different end users have different requirements for the CBUs requested? i.e., TNCs, processing needs, differences between your researchers versus your clinicians.
    - Do you request any testing be done by the CBB at the time of withdrawal? Do you conduct any testing when the CBB arrives at the hospital? Are CBUs discarded at this point for any reason?
    - Are you aware of how long a CBU is typically stored before it is withdrawn? Does this matter to you?
    - How often do you request a CBU? Do requests ever go unfulfilled? For what reasons? [*Clarify unfulfilled transplant versus research requests.*]

- Describe the chain of custody once a CBU arrives at your hospital.

- What quality checks are in place to ensure appropriate storage conditions before the CBU is used?

- [*If not already clear*] What works well about the current arrangements for obtaining a CBU? What problems exist? What changes would you make to the current system?

Contract Costs and Payments:

We are interested in learning about the economics of CBBs.

- How much do you typically pay for one CBU for research?
- How much do you typically pay for one CBU for transplant? Does the hospital pay and get reimbursed by payers, or does the CBB get reimbursed directly from the payer?
- How do cost considerations play a role in the decision to use CBUs versus other options for treatment? For research?
- At what point in the process is payment made? (e.g., at withdrawal only)
- What is the structure of payment arrangements between your organization and CBBs? A single payment per unit? Per-unit payment? Some combination of the two? Something else?
- Are there factors that influence the amount of payment? (i.e., does payment amount differ based on the payer?)
- Does payment amount differ based on CBU factors (TNC count, quality, HLA type, use [transplant versus research]) or other factors?
- Do you feel that your organization adequately compensates CBBs for cord blood? Why or why not? Do you have concerns about this going forward in the future?

Health Care System Trends

- Are there any innovations that may change the market significantly for your organization's use of cord blood? [*Potential probes: regenerative medicine, cell expansion for CBUs, use of double cords, etc.*]
- What trends or developments in the health care system are you worried about or have the potential to negatively impact your organization's use of CBUs?
  - [*Probe on affordable care organizations, global payments, Affordable Care Act coverage expansion, medical device excise tax, consolidation of hospital markets, regulatory requirements.*]

- Do you have any plans to make changes (e.g., business practices) to address these threats? If yes, please describe. What about your industry more broadly—are others making changes?
- What trends or developments in the health care system are you excited about? What trends or developments have the potential to positively impact your business?
  - [*Probe on affordable care organizations, global payments, Affordable Care Act coverage expansion, medical device excise tax, consolidation of hospital markets.*]

- Do you have any plans to make changes (e.g., business practices) to take better advantage of these opportunities? If yes, please describe. What about your industry more broadly— are others making changes?

–   We are thinking about how to improve the sustainability of the U.S. cord blood system. Do you have any concerns about the sustainability of the system as it currently exists or any recommendations to improve how cord blood is managed?

Appendix B. Economic Modeling

Here we present more details on how we derived our calculations in Chapter Seven. We estimated the value of CBUs based on their TNC count using aggregate NMDP data. As a starting point, consider a CBB that has some fixed inventory of CBUs that it wants to maintain, and is deciding on an appropriate TNC cut-off value to break even given this constraint. To calculate the TNC level at which the bank will achieve this, we need the following two equations for expected total revenue and expected total cost (Equations 1.1 and 1.2, respectively).

$$E[TR \mid TNC] = \sum_{I_0} P_i * (Fee - C_{dis}) + U(1 - d_1)(1 - d_2)(1 - d_3)S_B + U * S_c + \sum_{I_0} P_i S_s \qquad (1.1)$$

$$E[TC \mid TNC] = U(C_{coll} + (1 - d_1)C_{test} + (1 - d_1)(1 - d_2)(C_{pr} + C_s)) + I_0 C_s + Ad\min \qquad (1.2)$$

Where:

- P_i is the probability that unit i is chosen for transplant. It is a function of TNC count.
- *Fee* is the fee paid to the CBB by the transplanter or researcher.
- U is the average number of newly collected CBUs per year.
- I_0 is the initial bank-level inventory.
- d_1 is the preprocessing discard rate. It is a function of the TNC-count cut-off that banks choose and increasing in TNC.
- d_2 is the postprocessing discard rate and is constant.
- d_3 is the discard rate due to poor storage.
- $S_j, j = B, C, S$ are the subsidies that are paid for banking, collecting, and shipping (for NCBI CBUs only—about 60 percent of all banked units).
- C_k are the costs associated with each of the steps (k = coll [collection]; pr [processing]; test [testing]; s [storage]; dis [distribution]).
- *Ad* min are one-year CBBs' total overhead costs, such as equipment costs, maintenance contracts for equipment, rent, utilities, telephone, miscellaneous, office expenses, and labor costs.

These equations are based on the distribution of TNC counts across CBUs within the CBB and on the distribution of TNC counts in the population of CBUs, collected or not. The distribution of TNC counts within the CBB will be a truncation of the distribution of TNC counts within the population. The choice of the firm is to decide where to truncate the distribution. As a CBB increases the TNC cutoff for an acceptable unit, total costs rise because the probability of collecting an acceptable unit decreases. Alternatively, as the average TNC count of a unit with the bank increases, the probability that the unit will be shipped for transplant increases (see Chapter Seven for more details).

Parameters like Fee, d_2, d_3, C_k, and Ad min are exogenous to CBBs' decision on the TNC cut-off. We calculated and described most of these parameter values in the main report. We calculate Fee and C_k as the average from NMDP data and information obtained from our interviews with public CBBs, as well as published literature. Parameters d_2 and d_3 refer to postprocessing discard rates. We calculated them from data provided to us by one of the public CBBs that we interviewed. In Table B.1, we summarize these and other parameters used in this exercise.

Table B.1. Parameter Values and Sources

Parameter	Value	Source
Fee	$36,200	Interviews, NMDP data, other
d_2	0.25	Interviews
d_3	0.02	Interviews
C_{coll}	$200	Interviews, NMDP data, other
C_{test}	$700	Interviews, NMDP data, other
C_{pr}	$400	Interviews, NMDP data, other
C_S	$30	Interviews, NMDP data, other
C_{dis}	$720	NMDP data, other
Ad min	$2,376,462	NMDP data
I_0	18,282	Interviews, NMDP data
U	9,786	NMDP data

SOURCE: RAND authors' calculations.

Two other parameters, d_1 and P_i, are endogenous to CBBs' decision on TNC cut-off level because they both increase with CBU TNC count. To estimate d_1 and P_i by TNC count, we used the distribution of CBUs identified in Figure 6.2.[121] We assumed that the distribution of TNC counts is log-normally distributed and estimate its mean and standard deviation. While Naing et al. do not provide information on individual data points, they provide information on the mean (1.086×10^9) and standard deviation (0.651×10^9) of their data.[121] This allowed us to estimate the log-normal preprocessing TNC-count distribution. First, we took 1,000 random draws from a normal distribution with mean 1.086×10^9 and standard deviation 0.651×10^9. Then we computed the mean, the standard deviation, and the natural logs of these draws. We assumed that the TNC-count distribution was log-normally distributed with mean 20.77 and standard deviation 0.625. We then calculated d_1 as the cumulative density function (CDF) of this distribution. In Table B.1, we estimated probabilities that the collected CBU will be below a certain TNC value, which in turn helped us calculate an estimate for d_1 by TNC-count bins (see Table B.2). We used this CDF to develop the distribution of TNC counts within the bank so that we can estimate the probability that a CBU with a certain TNC level falls within different TNC bins.

Table B.2. Discretized CDF of TNC Counts

TNC (10^9)	CDF
Less than 0.90	0.40
Less than 1.25	0.61
Less than 1.50	0.73
Less than 1.75	0.79
Less than 2.00	0.85
Less than 2.50	0.92
Less than 3.00	0.95

SOURCE: RAND authors' calculations.

From these probabilities, we constructed the distribution of units for all potential cut-offs and calculated probabilities that a CBU will be banked given the TNC cut-off.

Appendix C. Donor Race/Ethnicity Matches

Table C.1. Percentage of Patient–Donor Race/Ethnicity Matches, by TNC Count

Patient	Donor				
	African-American	Asian/Pacific Islander	Caucasian	Hispanic	Other
Overall: All TNC Counts					
African-American	42.40%	1.10%	32.00%	0.60%	23.90%
Asian/Pacific Islander	1.40%	37.70%	36.70%	0.30%	23.90%
Caucasian	3.00%	1.60%	72.90%	0.60%	21.90%
Hispanic	9.10%	0.00%	90.90%	0.00%	0.00%
Other	8.90%	3.80%	68.10%	0.90%	18.30%
TNC: Less than 0.9×10^9					
African-American	53.1%	6.30%	21.90%	0.00%	18.80%
Asian/Pacific Islander	0.00%	61.10%	16.70%	0.00%	22.20%
Caucasian	8.00%	3.40%	49.4%	1.10%	37.90%
Hispanic	0.00%	0.00%	0.00%	0.00%	0.00%
Other	23.70%	7.50%	45.20%	4.30%	19.40%
TNC: $0.9–1.24 \times 10^9$					
African-American	58.70%	0.60%	16.20%	1.20%	23.40%
Asian/Pacific Islander	3.40%	57.50%	24.10%	0.00%	14.90%
Caucasian	4.60%	2.60%	74.20%	1.20%	17.30%
Hispanic	33.30%	0.00%	66.70%	0.00%	0.00%
Other	10.90%	6.30%	67.10%	2.00%	13.70%
TNC: $1.25–1.49 \times 10^9$					
African-American	45.40%	1.50%	30.10%	0.00%	23.00%
Asian/Pacific Islander	1.10%	45.50%	31.80%	0.00%	21.60%
Caucasian	4.30%	1.90%	75.50%	0.90%	17.40%
Hispanic	0.00%	0.00%	100.00%	0.00%	0.00%
Other	10.00%	6.50%	66.60%	0.70%	16.30%
TNC: $1.50–1.74 \times 10^9$					
African-American	42.70%	0.90%	31.50%	1.70%	23.30%
Asian/Pacific Islander	0.90%	31.60%	43.90%	0.00%	23.70%
Caucasian	2.70%	2.40%	73.50%	0.90%	20.60%
Hispanic	0.00%	0.00%	100.00%	0.00%	0.00%
Other	8.50%	3.80%	70.80%	0.40%	16.40%

TNC: More than $1.75×10^9$					
African-American	37.00%	0.90%	37.20%	0.30%	24.70%
Asian/Pacific Islander	1.20%	31.20%	39.90%	0.60%	27.00%
Caucasian	2.50%	1.10%	72.70%	0.40%	23.30%
Hispanic	0.00%	0.00%	100.00%	0.00%	0.00%
Other	7.50%	2.30%	69.20%	0.60%	20.30%

SOURCE: RAND authors' calculations using NMDP data for matches between donors and patients over the period 2010–2016.
NOTE: Patterns are similar for other races/ethnicities.

References

1. U.S. Government Accountability Office. National Cord Blood Inventory: Practices for Increasing Availability for Transplants and Related Challenges. Washington, DC; 2011:34.

2. King A, Shenoy S. Evidence-based focused review of the status of hematopoietic stem cell transplantation as treatment of sickle cell disease and thalassemia. Blood. 2014;123(20):3089-3094.

3. Hsieh MM, Fitzhugh CD, Tisdale JF. Allogeneic hematopoietic stem cell transplantation for sickle cell disease: the time is now. Blood. 2011;118(5):1197-1207.

4. Higgs DR. A new dawn for stem-cell therapy. The New England Journal of Medicine. 2008;358(9):964.

5. Fulco I, Miot S, Haug MD, et al. Engineered autologous cartilage tissue for nasal reconstruction after tumour resection: an observational first-in-human trial. The Lancet. 2014;384(9940):337-346.

6. Hirt MN, Hansen A, Eschenhagen T. Cardiac Tissue Engineering. Circulation Research. 2014;114(2):354-367.

7. Gratwohl A, Pasquini MC, Aljurf M, et al. One million haemopoietic stem-cell transplants: a retrospective observational study. The Lancet Haematology. 2015;2(3):e91-e100.

8. Rubinstein P. Why cord blood? Human Immunology. 2006;67(6):398-404.

9. Regan D. The power & potential of cord blood. Heart of America Association of Blood Banks. 2014; http://www.haabb.org/images/06-HAABB_2013_no_notes.pdf. Accessed August 17, 2017.

10. Niederwieser D, Baldomero H, Szer J, et al. Hematopoietic stem cell transplantation activity worldwide in 2012 and a SWOT analysis of the Worldwide Network for Blood and Marrow Transplantation Group including the global survey. Bone Marrow Transplantation. 2016.

11. National Cancer Institute. Cancer Stat Facts: Acute Myeloid Leukemia (AML). 2017; https://seer.cancer.gov/statfacts/html/amyl.html. Accessed August 10, 2017.

12. National Cancer Institute. Cancer Stat Facts: Acute Lymphocytic Leukemia (ALL). 2017; https://seer.cancer.gov/statfacts/html/alyl.html. Accessed August 10, 2017.

13.   Wingo PA, Cardinez CJ, Landis SH, et al. Long-term trends in cancer mortality in the United States, 1930–1998. Cancer. 2003;97(S12):3133-3275.

14.   Greenlee RT, Hill-Harmon MB, Murray T, Thun M. Cancer statistics, 2001. CA: A Cancer Journal for Clinicians. 2001;51(1):15-36.

15.   Horowitz MM. Trends in Graft Sources for Allogenic Hematopoietic Stem Cell Transplantation (HCT): Everyone Has a Donor. HRSA Advisory Council on Blood Stem Cell Transplantation Meetings; Rockville, MD; September 2016.

16.   Barker JN, Byam CE, Kernan NA, et al. Availability of cord blood extends allogeneic hematopoietic stem cell transplant access to racial and ethnic minorities. Biology of Blood and Marrow Transplantation. 2010;16(11):1541-1548.

17.   HLA Matching. 2016; https://bethematch.org/for-patients-and-families/ finding-a-donor/hla-matching. Accessed February 24, 2017.

18.   Human leukocyte antigens. Genetics Home Reference. 2009; https://ghr.nlm.nih.gov/primer/genefamily/hla. Accessed February 24, 2017.

19.   Madureira ABM, Eapen M, Locatelli F, et al. Analysis of risk factors influencing outcome in children with myelodysplastic syndrome after unrelated cord blood transplantation. Leukemia. 2011;25(3):449-454.

20.   A Comparison of Stem Cell Sources: Key Differences in Therapeutic Viability and Effectiveness. Stem Cells: Under the Microscope. 2007; https://www.cordblood.com/ about-cbr/stem-cell-information/march-2007. Accessed February 24, 2017.

21.   Magalon J, Maiers M, Kurtzberg J, et al. Banking or bankrupting: strategies for sustaining the economic future of public cord blood banks. PloS One. 2015;10(12):e0143440.

22.   Bone Marrow Donors Worldwide. A global database of lifesaving stem cell donors. 2017; https://www.bmdw.org. Accessed December 30, 2016.

23.   Cryo-Save. Cord Blood By Numbers. Date unknown; https://parentsguidecordblood.org/ sites/default/files/uploaded-files/infographic_cryo-save-sa.pdf. Accessed December 30, 2016.

24.   Institute of Medicine. Cord Blood: Establishing a National Hematopoietic Stem Cell Bank Program. Washington, DC: The National Academies Press; 2005.

25.   Ballen K, Verter F, Kurtzberg J. Umbilical cord blood donation: public or private? Bone Marrow Transplantation. 2015;50(10):1271-1278.

26.   Thornley I, Eapen M, Sung L, Lee SJ, Davies SM, Joffe S. Private cord blood banking: experiences and views of pediatric hematopoietic cell transplantation physicians. Pediatrics. 2009;123(3):1011-1017.

27.   Fisk N, Atun R. Public-private partnership in cord blood banking. BMJ: British Medical Journal. 2008;336(7645):642-644.

28.   U.S. Food and Drug Administration. Biologics Establishment Registration. 2011; http://www.fda.gov/BiologicsBloodVaccines/GuidanceComplianceRegulatoryInformation/EstablishmentRegistration. Accessed December 30, 2016.

29.   Be The Match.org. Participating Hospitals. 2017; https://bethematch.org/support-the-cause/donate-cord-blood/how-to-donate-cord-blood/participating-hospitals. Accessed June 26, 2017.

30.   Cordbloodawareness.org. Cord Blood Legislation: State by State. 2016; http://cordbloodawareness.org/state_legislation.htm. Accessed December 30, 2016.

31.   U.S. Food and Drug Administration. CFR—Code of Federal Regulations Title 21. 2016; http://www.accessdata.fda.gov/scripts/cdrh/cfdocs/cfcfr/CFRSearch.cfm?CFRPart=1271. Accessed December 30, 2016.

32.   Broder SM, Ponsaran RS, Goldenberg AJ. US public cord blood banking practices: recruitment, donation, and the timing of consent. Transfusion. 2013;53(3):679-687.

33.   Wada RK, Bradford A, Moogk M, et al. Cord blood units collected at a remote site: a collaborative endeavor to collect umbilical cord blood through the Hawaii Cord Blood Bank and store the units at the Puget Sound Blood Center. Transfusion. 2004;44(1):111-118.

34.   New York Blood Center. NCBP at Work: Processing, Freezing, Storage & Testing. 2015; http://www.nationalcordbloodprogram.org/work/process_test_storage.html. Accessed December 30, 2016.

35.   Blood AAo. Donor Eligibility (Screening and Testing). Date unknown; http://www.aabb.org/advocacy/regulatorygovernment/ct/hctps/de/Pages/default.aspx. Accessed December 30, 2016.

36.   Program NMD. NMDP Current Inventory Requirements for New Cord Blood Units. 2012.

37.   Peplow T. Public Cord Blood Banking in the U.S.: Business Models, Sustainability and Future Possibilities. 2013; http://www.totalbiopharma.com/2013/10/01/public-cord-blood-banking-business-models-sustainability-future-possibilities. Accessed December 30, 2016.

38.   New York Blood Center. NCBP at Work: Finding a Match. 2015; http://www.nationalcordbloodprogram.org/work/finding_a_match.html. Accessed December 30, 2016.

39.   BeTheMatch.org. Global Transplant Network. 2016; https://bethematch.org/about-us/global-transplant-network. Accessed December 30, 2016.

40.   Eapen M. HLA Match Likelihoods For Hematopoietic Stem-Cell Grafts in the US Registry. HRSA Advisory Council on Blood Stem Cell Transplantation (ACBSCT); Rockville, MD; September 15, 2014.

41.   BeTheMatch.org. Transplant Basics. 2017; https://bethematch.org/transplant-basics. Accessed February 24, 2017.

42.   Gyurkocza B, Sandmaier BM. Conditioning regimens for hematopoietic cell transplantation: one size does not fit all. Blood. 2014;124(3):344-353.

43.   BeTheMatch.org. Engraftment: Days 0–30. 2017; https://bethematch.org/for-patients-and-families/getting-a-transplant/engraftment--days-0-30. Accessed June 23, 2017.

44.   Ballen KK, Joffe S, Brazauskas R, et al. Hospital length of stay in the first 100 days after allogeneic hematopoietic cell transplantation for acute leukemia in remission: comparison among alternative graft sources. Biology of Blood and Marrow Transplantation. 2014;20(11):1819-1827.

45.   Stem Cell Therapeutic and Research Act of 2005. 119 STAT. 109th Congress; ed2005:2550-2563.

46.   Stem Cell Therapeutic and Research Reauthorization Act of 2010. 124 STAT. 111th Congress; ed2010:2789-2794.

47.   Stem Cell Therapeutic and Research Reauthorization Act of 2015. HR 2820. 114th Congress; ed2015.

48.   Health Resources and Services Administration. National Cord Blood Inventory Program Contractors. 2017; https://bloodcell.transplant.hrsa.gov/about/contractors/ncbi/index.html. Accessed May 31, 2017.

49.   Wabeke A. HRSA Requirements for Cord Blood Bank Accreditation. HRSA Advisory Council on Blood Stem Cell Transplantation Meetings; Rockville, MD; March 3, 2016.

50.   AABB Accredited Cord Blood (CB) Facilities. 2017; http://www.aabb.org/sa/facilities/celltherapy/Pages/CordBloodAccrFac.aspx. Accessed June 2, 2017.

51.   Foundation for the Accreditation of Cellular Therapy. 2017; http://www.factwebsite.org. Accessed June 2, 2017.

52.   Standards and Accreditation FAQs. 2017; http://www.aabb.org/sa/Pages/standards-accreditation-faqs.aspx. Accessed February 24, 2017.

53. Establishing Global Standards in Cellular Therapies. 2014; http://www.factwebsite.org/standards. Accessed February 24, 2017.

54. McCullough J. Workgroup Cord Blood Thawing and Washing Charge/Accomplishments/Next Steps. HRSA Advisory Council on Blood Stem Cell Transplantation (ACBSCT); Rockville, MD; May 29, 2014.

55. WMDA. WMDA Accreditation Programme. https://www.wmda.info/professionals/accreditation. Accessed December 30, 2016.

56. Laughlin MJ. Cleveland Cord Blood Center Biologics License Application (BLA). Advisory Council on Blood Stem Cell Transplantation Meetings; Rockville, MD; September 15, 2014.

57. Todd D. Bergen Community Regional Blood Center, Inc. HRSA Advisory Council on Blood Stem Cell Transplantation Meetings; Rockville, MD; September 15, 2014.

58. Kurtzberg J. Impact of FDA Licensure on Cord Blood Banking and Transplantation. HRSA Advisory Council on Blood Stem Cell Transplantation Meetings; Rockville, MD; May 29, 2014.

59. Freed BM. FDA Licensed Cord Blood Banking. HRSA Advisory Council on Blood Stem Cell Transplantation Meetings; Rockville, MD; May 29, 2014.

60. St. Louis Cord Blood Bank. HRSA Advisory Council on Blood Stem Cell Transplantation Meetings; May 29, 2014, Impact of FDA Licensure on Cord Blood Banking & Transplantation; Rockville, MD; May 29, 2014.

61. U.S. Food and Drug Administration. Cellular and Gene Therapy Products. Vaccines, Blood & Biologics. 2017; http://www.fda.gov/BiologicsBloodVaccines/CellularGeneTherapyProducts/ApprovedProducts/default.htm. Accessed February 24, 2017.

62. Bersenev A. FDA licenses first cord blood product. 2011. http://stemcellassays.com/2011/11/fda-licenses-cord-blood-product. Accessed August 10, 2017.

63. U.S. Food and Drug Administration. Cord Blood Banking—Information for Consumers. 2012; http://www.fda.gov/BiologicsBloodVaccines/ResourcesforYou/Consumers/ucm236044.htm. Accessed December 30, 2016.

64. U.S. Food and Drug Administration. Investigational New Drug Applications (INDs) for Minimally Manipulated, Unrelated Allogeneic Placental/Umbilical Cord Blood Intended for Hematopoietic Reconstitution for Specified Indications. 2011; http://www.fda.gov/downloads/BiologicsBloodVaccines/GuidanceComplianceRegulatoryInformation/Guidances/Blood/UCM266021.pdf. Accessed December 30, 2016.

65. World Marrow Donor Association. Database. 2017; https://share.wmda.info/display/WMDAREG/Database. Accessed June 9, 2017.

66. Patton MQ. Qualitative Research. Encyclopedia of Statistics in Behavioral Science, John Wiley & Sons, Ltd.; 2005.

67. Bradley EH, Curry LA, Devers KJ. Qualitative data analysis for health services research: developing taxonomy, themes, and theory. Health Services Research. 2007;42(4):1758-1772.

68. Miles M, Huberman A. Qualitative Data Analysis: An Expanded Sourcebook. Thousand Oaks, CA: Sage Publications; 1994.

69. Ryan G, Bernard H. Techniques to Identify Themes. Field Methods. 2003;15(1):85-109.

70. FDA Center for Biologics Evaluation and Research. Human Cell and Tissue Establishment Registration: Public Query Enter Query Criteria. 2016; https://www.accessdata.fda.gov/scripts/cber/CFAppsPub/tiss/index.cfm. Accessed August 10, 2017.

71. Request for Information: National Cord Blood Inventory. 2013; https://www.fbo.gov/index?s=opportunity&mode=form&id=6f3269f0a7a975c5bba6a4ac265 67cb0&tab=core&_cview=0. Accessed August 10, 2017.

72. Healthcare Cost and Utilization Project. HCUP Databases. 2017; http://www.hcup-us.ahrq.gov/nisoverview.jsp. Accessed June 6, 2017.

73. Fryar CD, Gu Q, Ogden CL. Anthropometric reference data for children and adults: United States, 2007–2010. Vital and Health Statistics Series 11, Data from the National Health Survey. 2012(252):1-48.

74. Committee on Obstetric Practice. ACOG committee opinion number 399, February 2008: umbilical cord blood banking. Obstetrics and Gynecology. 2008;111(2 Pt 1):475.

75. American Academy of Pediatrics. Delayed Umbilical Cord Clamping After Birth. Pediatrics. 2017;139(6):e20170957.

76. American College of Obstetricians and Gynecologists. Delayed umbilical cord clamping after birth. Obstetrics and Gynecology. 2017;129:e5-10.

77. Grant S. Program Report to the Advisory Council on Blood Stem Cell Transplantation. Paper presented at: HRSA Advisory Council on Blood Stem Cell Transplantation (ACBSCT); Rockville, MD; September 11, 2015; https://bloodcell.transplant.hrsa.gov/about/advisory_council/meetings/programreportadvisory councilbloodstemcelltransplantation.pdf. Accessed September 22, 2017.

78.   Todd D. Why Is Cord Blood Banking So Expensive? 2012;
        https://parentsguidecordblood.org/en/news/why-cord-blood-banking-so-expensive. Accessed
        June 14, 2017.

79.   Wagner JE, Barker JN, DeFor TE, et al. Transplantation of unrelated donor umbilical
        cord blood in 102 patients with malignant and nonmalignant diseases: influence of CD34 cell
        dose and HLA disparity on treatment-related mortality and survival. Blood.
        2002;100(5):1611-1618.

80.   Jones J, Stevens CE, Rubinstein P, Robertazzi RR, Kerr A, Cabbad MF. Obstetric
        predictors of placental/umbilical cord blood volume for transplantation. American Journal of
        Obstetrics and Gynecology. 2003;188(2):503-509.

81.   Lauber S, Latta M, Klüter H, Müller-Steinhardt M. The Mannheim cord blood bank:
        experiences and perspectives for the future. Transfusion Medicine and Hemotherapy.
        2010;37(2):90-97.

82.   Lecchi L, Ratti I, Lazzari L, Rebulla P, Sirchia G. Reasons for discard of umbilical cord
        blood units before cryopreservation. Transfusion. 2000;40(1):122-123.

83.   Stem Cell Therapeutic and Research Act of 2005. Smith RCH, trans. 109th ed. 2005.

84.   BioBridge Global. 2015 Annual Report. 2015;
        https://gencure.org/sites/default/files/2015_annual-report_prweb_site.pdf Accessed
        September 22, 2017.

85.   Complete 2015-16 Global Cord Blood Banking. 2016;
        http://www.bioinformant.com/product/complete-2015-16-global-cord-blood-banking-
        industry-report. Accessed December 2, 2016.

86.   Howard DH, Meltzer D, Kollman C, et al. Use of cost-effectiveness analysis to determine
        inventory size for a national cord blood bank. Medical Decision Making. 2008;28(2):243-
        253.

87.   Cord Blood Education Legislation. Date unknown; http://www.cordblood.com/benefits-
        cord-blood/umbilical-cord-blood-banking/cord-blood-banking-legislation. Accessed August
        17, 2017.

88.   Form 990: Return of Organization Exempt from Income Tax: The Cleveland Foundation.
        In: Internal Revenue Service, ed2014.

89.   Khera N, Zeliadt SB, Lee SJ. Economics of hematopoietic cell transplantation. Blood.
        2012;120(8):1545-1551.

90.   Couban S, Dranitsaris G, Andreou P, et al. Clinical and economic analysis of allogeneic peripheral blood progenitor cell transplants: a Canadian perspective. Bone Marrow Transplantation. 1998;22(12):1199-1205.

91.   Saito A, Zahrieh D, Cutler C, et al. Lower costs associated with hematopoietic cell transplantation using reduced intensity vs high-dose regimens for hematological malignancy. Bone Marrow Transplantation. 2007;40(3):209-217.

92.   Saito AM, Cutler C, Zahrieh D, et al. Costs of allogeneic hematopoietic cell transplantation with high-dose regimens. Biology of Blood and Marrow Transplantation. 2008;14(2):197-207.

93.   Rizzo JD, Vogelsang GB, Krumm S, Frink B, Mock V, Bass EB. Outpatient-based bone marrow transplantation for hematologic malignancies: cost saving or cost shifting? Journal of Clinical Oncology. 1999;17(9):2811-2811.

94.   Svahn B-M, Alvin O, Ringdén O, Gardulf A, Remberger M. Costs of allogeneic hematopoietic stem cell transplantation. Transplantation. 2006;82(2):147-153.

95.   Majhail NS, Mothukuri JM, Brunstein CG, Weisdorf DJ. Costs of hematopoietic cell transplantation: comparison of umbilical cord blood and matched related donor transplantation and the impact of posttransplant complications. Biology of Blood and Marrow Transplantation. 2009;15(5):564-573.

96.   Cordonnier C, Maury S, Esperou H, et al. Do minitransplants have minicosts? A cost comparison between myeloablative and nonmyeloablative allogeneic stem cell transplant in patients with acute myeloid leukemia. Bone Marrow Transplantation. 2005;36(7):649-654.

97.   Advisory Council on Blood Stem Cell Transplantation. ACBSCT Update on Medicare Reimbursement Initiatives. Rockville, MD; 2016.

98.   Costa V, McGregor M, Laneuville P, Brophy JM. The cost-effectiveness of stem cell transplantations from unrelated donors in adult patients with acute leukemia. Value Health. 2007;10(4):247-255.

99.   Lin Y-F, Lairson DR, Chan W, et al. The costs and cost-effectiveness of allogeneic peripheral blood stem cell transplantation versus bone marrow transplantation in pediatric patients with acute leukemia. Biology of Blood and Marrow Transplantation. 2010;16(9):1272-1281.

100.   Matthes-Martin S, Pötschger U, Barr R, et al. Costs and cost-effectiveness of allogeneic stem cell transplantation in children are predictable. Biology of Blood and Marrow Transplantation. 2012;18(10):1533-1539.

135

101.   Majhail NS, Mau L-W, Denzen EM, Arneson TJ. Costs of autologous and allogeneic hematopoietic cell transplantation in the United States: a study using a large national private claims database. Bone Marrow Transplantation. 2013;48(2):294-300.

102.   Dix SP, Geller RB. High-dose chemotherapy with autologous stem cell rescue in the outpatient setting. Oncology. 2000;14(2):171-185; discussion 185-176, 191-172.

103.   Majhail NS, Mau L-W, Payton T, Denzen EM. National Survey of Blood and Marrow Transplant Center Personnel, Infrastructure and Models of Care Delivery. Center for International Blood and Marrow Transplant Research; February 1, 2015.

104.   Preussler JM, Farnia SH, Denzen EM, Majhail NS. Variation in Medicaid coverage for hematopoietic cell transplantation. Journal of Oncology Practice. 2014;10(4):e196-e200.

105.   Centers for Medicare and Medicaid Services. National Coverage Determination (NCD) for Stem Cell Transplantation (110.8.1). Vol 100-32010.

106.   Centers for Medicare and Medicaid Services. Proposed National Coverage Determination for Stem Cell Transplantation (Multiple Myeloma, Myelofibrosis, and Sickle Cell Disease) (CAG-00444R). 2015.

107.   Centers for Medicare and Medicaid Services, U.S. Department of Health and Human Services. Acute Care Hospital Inpatient Prospective Payment System. ICN 006815; December 2016; https://www.cms.gov/Outreach-and-Education/Medicare-Learning-Network-MLN/MLNProducts/downloads/AcutePaymtSysfctsht.pdf. Accessed August 17, 2017.

108.   Centers for Medicare and Medicaid Services. Draft ICD-10-CM/PCS MS-DRGv28 Definitions Manual: Pre-MDC Allogenic Bone Marrow Transplant. Date unknown; https://www.cms.gov/icd10manual/fullcode_cms/P0043.html. Accessed August 10, 2017.

109.   UnitedHealthCare. Umbilical Cord Blood Harvesting for Storage and Future Use. UnitedHealthCare Commercial Medical Policy. 2016.

110.   Annas GJ. Waste and longing—the legal status of placental-blood banking. Massachusetts Medical Society. 1999.

111.   Moise Jr KJ. Umbilical cord stem cells. Obstetrics and Gynecology. 2005;106(6):1393-1407.

112.   Majhail NS, Omondi NA, Denzen E, Murphy EA, Rizzo JD. Access to hematopoietic cell transplantation in the United States. Biology of Blood and Marrow Transplantation. 2010;16(8):1070-1075.

113. Mitchell JM, Meehan KR, Kong J, Schulman KA. Access to bone marrow transplantation for leukemia and lymphoma: the role of sociodemographic factors. Journal of Clinical Oncology. 1997;15(7):2644-2651.

114. Blood and Marrow Transplant Clinical Trials Network. BMT CTN Protocol 1101. 2017; https://web.emmes.com/study/bmt2/protocol/1101_protocol/1101_protocol.html. Accessed June 28, 2017.

115. Brunstein CG, Laughlin MJ. Extending cord blood transplant to adults: dealing with problems and results overall. Seminars in Hematology. 2010;47(1):86-96.

116. Laughlin MJ, Eapen M, Rubinstein P, et al. Outcomes after transplantation of cord blood or bone marrow from unrelated donors in adults with leukemia. New England Journal of Medicine. 2004;351(22):2265-2275.

117. Rocha V, Labopin M, Sanz G, et al. Transplants of umbilical-cord blood or bone marrow from unrelated donors in adults with acute leukemia. New England Journal of Medicine. 2004;351(22):2276-2285.

118. Milano F, Gooley T, Wood B, et al. Cord-blood transplantation in patients with minimal residual disease. New England Journal of Medicine. 2016;375(10):944-953.

119. Eapen M, Rubinstein P, Zhang MJ, et al. Outcomes of transplantation of unrelated donor umbilical cord blood and bone marrow in children with acute leukaemia: a comparison study. Lancet (London, England). 2007;369(9577):1947-1954.

120. Takahashi S, Ooi J, Tomonari A, et al. Comparative single-institute analysis of cord blood transplantation from unrelated donors with bone marrow or peripheral blood stem-cell transplants from related donors in adult patients with hematologic malignancies after myeloablative conditioning regimen. Blood. 2007;109(3):1322-1330.

121. Naing MW, Gibson DA, Hourd P, et al. Improving umbilical cord blood processing to increase total nucleated cell count yield and reduce cord input wastage by managing the consequences of input variation. Cytotherapy. 2015;17(1):58-67.

122. Shlebak A, Roberts I, Stevens T, Szydlo R, Goldman J, Gordon M. The impact of antenatal and perinatal variables on cord blood haemopoietic stem/progenitor cell yield available for transplantation. British Journal of Haematology. 1998;103:1167-1171.

123. George TJ, Sugrue MW, George SN, Wingard JR. Factors associated with parameters of engraftment potential of umbilical cord blood. Transfusion. 2006;46(10):1803-1812.

124. Cobellis L, Castaldi M, Trabucco E, et al. Cord blood unit bankability can be predicted by prenatal sonographic parameters. European Journal of Obstetrics and Gynecology and Reproductive Biology. 2013;170(2):391-395.

125. Jamali M, Atarodi K, Nakhlestani M, et al. Cord blood banking activity in Iran National Cord Blood Bank: A two years experience. Transfusion and Apheresis Science. 2014;50(1):129-135.

126. Keersmaekers CL, Mason BA, Keersmaekers J, Ponzini M, Mlynarek RA. Factors affecting umbilical cord blood stem cell suitability for transplantation in an in-utero collection program. Transfusion. 2014;54(3):545-549.

127. Bart T, Boo M, Balabanova S, et al. Impact of selection of cord blood units from the United States and Swiss registries on the cost of banking operations. Transfusion Medicine and Hemotherapy. 2013;40(1):14-20.

128. Lee Y-H, Kim JY, Mun Y-C, Koo HH. A proposal for improvement in the utilization rate of banked cord blood. Blood Research. 2013;48(1):5-7.

129. Clark P, Elwood N, Rodwell R, Holdsworth R, Montague A. Analysis of the Australian cord blood (CB) inventory and collection and banking strategies. 9th Annual International Cord Blood Transplantation Symposium; San Francisco, CA; 2011.

130. Brown N, Machin L, McLeod D. Immunitary bioeconomy: the economisation of life in the international cord blood market. Social Science and Medicine. 2011;72(7):1115-1122.

131. Wang TF, Wen SH, Yang KL, et al. Reasons for exclusion of 6,820 umbilical cord blood donations in a public cord blood bank. Transfusion. 2014;54(1):231-237.

132. Askari S, Miller J, Chrysler G, McCullough J. Impact of donor-and collection-related variables on product quality in ex utero cord blood banking. Transfusion. 2005;45(2):189-194.

133. Yessian MR, Hereford RW, Robboy E, Levine A. National Marrow Donor Program: Progress in Minority Recruitment. In: U.S. Department of Health and Human Services Office of Inspector General, ed. Boston, MA; 1996.

134. Katz G. Industrial Economics of Cord Blood Banks. Cord Blood Stem Cells and Regenerative Medicine, Elsevier; 2015:325-345.

135. Advisory Council on Blood Stem Cell Transplantation. Meeting Minutes. Paper presented at: Advisory Council on Blood Stem Cell Transplantation; Rockville, MD; March 3, 2016.

136. Ballen KK, Hicks J, Dharan B, et al. Racial and ethnic composition of volunteer cord blood donors: comparison with volunteer unrelated marrow donors. Transfusion. 2002;42(10):1279-1284.

137. Tossounian SA, Schoendorf KC, Kiely JL. Racial differences in perceived barriers to prenatal care. Maternal and Child Health Journal. 1997;1(4):229-236.

138. Ballen KK, Kurtzberg J, Lane TA, et al. Racial diversity with high nucleated cell counts and CD34 counts achieved in a national network of cord blood banks. Biology of Blood and Marrow Transplantation. 2004;10(4):269-275.

139. Akyurekli C, Chan J, Elmoazzen H, Tay J, Allan DS. Impact of ethnicity on human umbilical cord blood banking: a systematic review. Transfusion. 2014;54(8):2122-2127.

140. Gragert L, Eapen M, Williams E, et al. HLA match likelihoods for hematopoietic stem-cell grafts in the U.S. registry. New England Journal of Medicine. 2014;371(4):339-348.

141. Barker JN, Scaradavou A, Stevens CE. Combined effect of total nucleated cell dose and HLA match on transplantation outcome in 1,061 cord blood recipients with hematologic malignancies. Blood. 2010;115(9):1843-1849.

142. Arrojo IP, Lamas Mdel C, Verdugo LP, et al. Trends in cord blood banking. Blood Transfusion. 2012;10(1):95-100.

143. Petrini C. Umbilical cord blood banking: from personal donation to international public registries to global bioeconomy. Journal of Blood Medicine. 2014;5:87.

144. Natera, Inc. Announces Launch of Evercord™ Cord Blood and Tissue Banking Service [press release]. San Carolos, CA, March 1, 2017.

145. Lifeforce Cryobanks. 2017; https://parentsguidecordblood.org/en/banks/lifeforce-cryobanks. Accessed June 15, 2017.

146. O'Connor M, Samuel G, Jordens C, Kerridge I. Umbilical cord blood banking: beyond the public-private divide. The Journal of Law, Medicine, and Ethics. 2012;19(3):512-516.

147. Jordens CF, Kerridge IH, Stewart CL, et al. Knowledge, beliefs, and decisions of pregnant Australian women concerning donation and storage of umbilical cord blood: a population-based survey. Birth. 2014;41(4):360-366.

148. Hildreth C. Cord blood market analysis—costs and structures for public donation. 2016; http://www.bioinformant.com/cord-blood-market-analysis-cost-structure-for-public-donation. Accessed December 2, 2016.

149. Hildreth C. Do you know the fastest growing cord blood banks, by revenue? 2016; http://www.bioinformant.com/do-you-know-the-fastest-growing-cord-blood-banks-by-revenue. Accessed August 17, 2017.

150. Martin P, Brown N, Turner A. Capitalizing hope: the commercial development of umbilical cord blood stem cell banking. New Genetics and Society. 2008;27(2):127-143.

151. Passweg J, Baldomero H, Bader P, et al. Use of haploidentical stem cell transplantation continues to increase: the 2015 European Society for Blood and Marrow Transplant activity survey report. Bone Marrow Transplantation. 2017.

152.	Hino M, Yamane T. Non-myeloablative or reduced intensity stem cell transplantation preparative regimens. Nihon Rinsho Japanese Journal of Clinical Medicine. 2003;61(9):1535-1541.

153.	Delaney C, Heimfeld S, Brashem-Stein C, Voorhies H, Manger RL, Bernstein ID. Notch-mediated expansion of human cord blood progenitor cells capable of rapid myeloid reconstitution. Nature Medicine. 2010;16(2):232-236.

154.	Walasek MA, van Os R, de Haan G. Hematopoietic stem cell expansion: challenges and opportunities. Annals of the New York Academy of Sciences. 2012;1266(1):138-150.

155.	Maxmen A. Lab-grown blood stem cells produced at last. Nature. 2017.

156.	Cutler DM, McClellan M. Is technological change in medicine worth it? Health Affairs. 2001;20(5):11-29.

157.	Vigdor ER. Coverage does matter: the value of health forgone by the uninsured. Hidden Costs, Value Lost: Uninsurance in America. 2003:129-169.

158.	Ubel PA, Hirth RA, Chernew ME, Fendrick AM. What is the price of life and why doesn't it increase at the rate of inflation? Archives of Internal Medicine. 2003;163(14):1637-1641.

159.	Barker JN, Byam C, Scaradavou A. How I treat: the selection and acquisition of unrelated cord blood grafts. Blood. 2011:117(8):2332-2339; https://www.ncbi.nlm.nih.gov/pubmed/21149636. Accessed September 22, 2017.

160.	National Cord Blood Inventory Augmentation, Fifth Cohort. In: Health Resources and Services Administration, ed. Rockville, MD: Office of Acquisitions Management and Policy; 2010.

161.	Thaler Richard H, Sunstein Cass R. Nudge: improving decisions about health, wealth, and happiness. New Haven, CT: Yale University Press; 2008.

162.	Johnson EJ, Goldstein D. Do defaults save lives? American Association for the Advancement of Science; 2003.

163.	Transplant Center Search Results. 2017; https://bethematch.org/tcdirectory/search/advanced. Accessed August 10, 2017.

164.	Barker JN, Krepski TP, DeFor TE, Davies SM, Wagner JE, Weisdorf DJ. Searching for unrelated donor hematopoietic stem cells: availability and speed of umbilical cord blood versus bone marrow. Biology of Blood and Marrow Transplantation. 2002;8(5):257-260.